英汉对照
ENGLISH–CHINESE

A Collection of Medical English Practical Writings

医务英语应用文集

（第 2 版）

主编 王文秀 王 颖

人民卫生出版社

图书在版编目（CIP）数据

英汉对照医务英语应用文集 / 王文秀，王颖主编
. —2 版 . —北京：人民卫生出版社，2020
ISBN 978-7-117-29786-8

Ⅰ.①英…　Ⅱ.①王…　②王…　Ⅲ.①医学 - 英语 -
应用文 - 写作　Ⅳ.①R

中国版本图书馆 CIP 数据核字（2020）第 023237 号

人卫智网	www.ipmph.com	医学教育、学术、考试、健康，
		购书智慧智能综合服务平台
人卫官网	www.pmph.com	人卫官方资讯发布平台

英汉对照医务英语应用文集
（第 2 版）

主　　编：王文秀　王　颖
出版发行：人民卫生出版社（中继线 010-59780011）
地　　址：北京市朝阳区潘家园南里 19 号
邮　　编：100021
E - mail：pmph @ pmph.com
购书热线：010-59787592　010-59787584　010-65264830
印　　刷：三河市潮河印业有限公司
经　　销：新华书店
开　　本：850×1168　1/32　印张：11.5
字　　数：298 千字
版　　次：2003 年 7 月第 1 版　2020 年 3 月第 2 版
　　　　　2020 年 3 月第 2 版第 1 次印刷（总第 3 次印刷）
标准书号：ISBN 978-7-117-29786-8
定　　价：48.00 元
打击盗版举报电话：010-59787491　E-mail：WQ @ pmph.com
质量问题联系电话：010-59787234　E-mail：zhiliang @ pmph.com

　　《英汉对照医务英语应用文集》一书自 2003 年出版以来颇受业界人士的重视和广大读者厚爱,数次重印,传播甚广。考虑到本书的时代性、标准性和可操作性,我们对本书进行了此次修订。

　　本次修订在保持原书"选材立足实用,针对我国的国情和医务工作者对外交流情况现状,择需编写"的前提下,力求突出以下 4 个方面的特点。

　　(1)详细介绍了各种常见医学英语应用文的写作格式、要求和语言特点:读者在医学英语应用文写作和翻译中,如求职、求学、访问、学术交流、科研合作书信、临床报告、病历、医学证明等医务文件的撰写时,均能在本书找到范例,以达到"他山之石,可以攻玉"之目的。

　　(2)实用性强:遵循精讲多练的原则,融理论与实践于一体。各章节的主体部分均为汉英对照具体实例。使读者在学习和模仿过程中逐步了解和掌握医学英语应用文的写作和翻译技巧。

　　(3)针对性强:本书第 1 版曾在医学院校本科生、研究生和在职医生培训班中使用,取得了较好的效果。经过数轮教学实践,对原书的章节结构、内容和文体进一步精选提炼,充实了大量新内容,使本书具有了更强的针对性。

　　(4)全书由清晰、浅易的中英文写成。突出了实用和多举范例的特点。所选范文既有英美作者的原始文本,又有中国学者的力作佳篇,贴近实际,读来亲切,易于学习。

　　王珩教授对本书进行了认真的审阅;吴晓光、冯永平和巴一等人士亦为本书的编写和修订工作提供了帮助,金港广告有限公司刘丽红女士担任本书文字录入工作,在此一并表示真挚的感谢。

期待修订后的《英汉对照医务英语应用文集(第2版)》能够为广大读者的医学英语学习提供更好的参考。

王文秀
2019 年 5 月
于承德医学院

近年来,随着对外开放政策的逐步落实和中国医药走向世界,赴我国就医、求医的外国人日益增多,同时我国医生出国进行医务活动亦日趋频繁。2001 年我国正式成为世贸组织的成员,医疗卫生界的国际交流范围必将进一步扩大,医务人员将有更多的场合需要借助英语进行对外联络、交流。医务英语应用文的重要性也日益凸显。

囿于中国以前的国情和传统的外语教学和学习模式,应用文这种文体并未为大多数学习英语者所掌握,其撰写和使用也主要局限于涉外部门。这种现象极大地制约了我国医务人员与外国有关部门和人员之间的交流活动。为打破这一"桎梏",笔者以多年来从事援外医务人员英语培训工作和外联工作所积累的资料为依据,编写了这本《英汉对照医务英语应用文集》。

本书选材立足实用,针对我国的国情和医务工作者对外交流情况的现状,择需编写。所选范文均以真实书信和医务文件为基础,并经由中英文专家逐字逐句地修改、订正和润色。英文部分具有较高的水准;中文部分在体现原文风格的同时,亦兼顾了现代汉语的行文特征。本书涉及范围较广,信函部分设定了百余个不同的专题,涉及到求职、出国进修,学术交流等各种不同的场景;医务文件部分则提供了从入院记录,病历到专用证明等一系列进行涉外医务活动时所需撰写的医务文件的范文。本书所收录的大量的具有不同风格的典型范文能够满足不同层次的读者的需求。闲暇时,阅读本书能熟悉、掌握各种应用文的写法,了解欧美国家的社交习俗;急用时,则可根据所处的具体场景,选出范文进行模拟套写。

　　本书的出版与笔者于 2001 年出版的《医务英语会话》形成姊妹卷,目的在于为医务工作者进行对外交流时提供一双有力的翅膀。

王文秀
2002 年

目 录

信函（Letter）

英文书信（English Letter）大致可分为事务信件（Business Letter）和私人信件（Private Letter）两大类。前者指单位与单位之间，或单位与个人之间，因接洽工作而来往的信件；后者指亲属、朋友之间的来往信件。由于英文书信涉及面广，用途极为广泛，故根据不同的作用和用途还可细分为社交书信（Social Letter）、业务书信（Business Letter）、私人书信（Private Letter），以及一些既属于事务书信又属于私人书信的专门书信（Special Letter），如表扬信（Letter of commendation and encouragement）、感谢信（Letter of thanks）等。

第一节　邀请信（Invitation）

在各种社交书信中，邀请信是最常见的一种，这类信应写明：

（1）邀请人的姓名。

（2）邀请的目的。

（3）邀请在外停留起止时间。

（4）被邀请人的费用负担问题。

有时，在结束语中也可写上一些向对方表示崇敬的词句。

1. 邀请代表团访问（An invitation to a delegation）

亲爱的 ××× 博士：

　　×× 医学院副院长 ××× 博士已向我转告了您有意于 11 月份访问 ×× 医学院一事。

　　×× 医学院非常高兴能向您和您的代表团发出邀请，并欢迎您在随同高等教育代表团访问中国期间来我校参观。

　　有关日程问题，请与 ××× 博士联系，他将为您安排活动日程，这样可使您的代表团对我们学校以及共同感兴趣的问题有一个透彻的了解。

　　我们将为您提供在承德期间的食宿和交通费。

　　　　　　　　　　　　　　　　　　　　　您的真诚的
　　　　　　　　　　　　　　　　　　　　　××× 博士

Sept. 12, 2016

…, Ph. D.
Chancellor
East Carolina University
Greenville, North Carolina 27834

Dear Dr. …,

　　Dr. …, vice president of … Medical College, has made me aware of your interest in visiting … Medical College in November.

　　… Medical College is happy to extend to you and your delegation an invitation to visit our institution during the course of your tour of institutions of higher education in China.

　　Please contact with Dr. … regarding your itinerary so that he can arrange a schedule of activities that will provide your delegation with a good understanding of our institution and areas of mutual interest.

We will plan also to provide you with food, lodging and transportation during your stay in Chengde.

Sincerely yours,
(Signature)
…, M.D.

2. 邀请考察(An invitation for investigation)

亲爱的 ×××博士:

十分抱歉没能及时给您回信,但我十分高兴地告诉您,新疆维吾尔自治区卫生厅已最后同意您和 ×××博士自费去和田参观。我代表承德市邀请您和 ×××博士在 2016 年 8 月 22 日第二届亚太甲状腺协会会议结束后来中国访问。

×××博士和 ×××博士将陪同您们一起去新疆首府乌鲁木齐,并安排您们去参观地方性克汀病病区。您们从乌鲁木齐回来时,我也结束了在东京的第七届国际内分泌学会会议,届时将在承德迎候您和 ×××博士来访。

我们还邀请您们到承德围场去考察另一个地方性甲状腺肿和神经性克汀病病区。

我们在北京将为您们安排一个小型聚会,与河北、河南、贵州以及内蒙古的同行们会晤,并讨论有关在防治地方性甲状腺肿和临床及实验性克汀病方面进行合作研究的前景。

我院将承担您和 ×××博士在京、承两地的食宿和交通费用。

盼望在东京见到您和 ×××博士。

您的真诚的
×××博士

June 22, 2016

Dr. ...

Division of Human Nutrition, CSIRO

Kintore Avenue, Adelaide

South Australia

Dear Dr. ...,

I apologize for writing to you so late, but am pleased to tell you that Xinjiang Autonomous District Public Health Bureau has finally sanctioned your and Dr. ... 's visit to Hetian at your own expense. I am authorized, on behalf of Chengde Municipality, to invite you and Dr. ... to visit China after the 2nd AOTA Meeting closed on August 22nd, 2016.

You will be accompanied by Dr. ... and Dr. ... to Urumqi, capital of Xinjiang. They will arrange for you to visit an area where you can observe endemic cretinism. When you return from Urumqi, I shall be back from the 7th IEA Congress in Tokyo and ready to welcome you and Dr. ... to Chengde.

You are also invited to visit Weichang of Chengde Municipality, another small endemic area of goiter and neurological type of cretinism.

We shall have a small gathering in Beijing for you to meet some of our colleagues from Hebei, Henan, Guizhou and Inner Mongolia, and to discuss future cooperative investigations in the field of goiter control and clinical and experimental cretinism.

Expenses, including board, lodging, and vehicle for you and Dr. ... in Beijing and Chengde will be borne by our college.

Looking forward to seeing you and Dr. ... in Tokyo.

Sincerely yours,

(Signature)

..., M.D.

3. 邀请参加年会（An invitation to attend an annual meeting）

亲爱的 ×××博士：

我十分荣幸地邀请您来承德参加将于 2016 年 1 月 27 日至 29 日在水晶宫饭店举行的河北眼外科学会第 12 届年会。

作为我们的贵宾，我们将为您提供返程机票及在承德期间的食宿费。

盼望着在承德见到您。

您的真诚的

×××

Oct. 18, 2015

..., M.D.

Dept. of Ophthalmology

Houston State Univ.

Houston, TX 70956

Dear Dr. ...,

It is my great pleasure to invite you to the 12th Annual Meeting of Hebei Association of Ophthalic Surgeons which will be held on Jan.27–29, 2016 at Crystal Palace Hotel in Chengde.

Since you will be our distinguished guest, it is our wish to provide for your return airfare and hotel accommodation in Chengde.

I look forward to seeing you in Chengde.

Sincerely yours,

(Signature)

...

4. 邀请参加学术会议（An invitation to attend an academic conference）

亲爱的 ××× 博士：

　　C.L. 休博士给我写信，推荐您在 2017 年 3 月 23 日至 25 日在承德举行的第九届中国神经外科会议上做报告。我们热诚地欢迎您参加这次盛会。从休博士的信中得知，您报告的题目是"脑囊虫病"，它是亚洲国家神经外科研讨会受欢迎的题目。您可用 10 分钟进行演讲，5 分钟进行讨论。官方语言是英语和法语，同声翻译工作由一组中国神经外科医生承担。

　　3 月 26 日我们还将召开另外一组会议，即第 3 届显微外科解剖年会。随信附上这两次会议的日程表。

　　我将给您寄去来承德的机票，并为您提供在承食宿。为了得到承德市外事办公室的批准，请将您的出生日期、目前职位、在华日程及着陆机场名称通知我。

　　盼望着 2017 年 3 月见到您。

　　顺致最良好的祝愿。

您的真诚的
×××

Dec. 26, 2016

…, M.D.
Dept. of Neurosurgery
Neurological Institute
Kyushu Univ.
Maidashi 3–1–1, Fukuoka 812
Japan

Dear Dr. …,

　　Dr. C. L. Hew has written to me recommending you as a speaker at the 9th Chinese Congress of Neurological Surgeons (CCNS), which will be held on March 23–25, 2017 in Chengde, China. You are cordially invited to participate in our meeting. According to Dr. Hew, the title of your lecture is "Cerebral Cysticercosis", a welcome topic to the seminar on Neurosurgery in Asian countries. The allotted time for your presentation is 10 minutes and 5 minutes for discussion. The official languages are English and French. Simultaneous translation, in both English and French, is provided by a group of Chinese neurosurgeons.

On March 26, 2017 we shall have another meeting, the 3rd Annual Seminar of the Microsurgical Anatomy. I enclose programs of both meetings.

I shall send you the tickets for your flight to Chengde and offer accommodations during your stay in Chengde. I must have permission from the Chengde Foreign affairs Office for your visit, and, therefore, please provide me with your date of birth, present position, itinerary in China, and the names of airports you want to use.

I am looking forward to seeing you in March, 2017.

With my best regards,

Sincerely yours,

(Signature)

...

*　　*　　*

亲爱的萨宾教授：

　　两年一次的武汉大学病毒性疾病学术大会将于 2016 年 7 月 29—2016 年 7 月 31 日举行第 10 届会议。大会组委会计划将这次会议办成国际会议，邀请一些著名的外国病毒学专家与会。大会的正式语言是汉语和英语。

据熊贞敏教授说，您对这次会议很感兴趣。组委会想请您参加，介绍您的新发现。

您的有关费用，包括纽约—武汉往返旅费、交通、住宿均由组委会支付。

请告诉我您成行的可能性，并请告知您的护照号码，以便寄上签证申请表。

收到您的同意赴会的信函，我们立即奉寄正式邀请书和其他资料。

您忠实的

向天明

病毒性疾病大会第 10 届主席

Dear Professor Sabin,

The Conference on "Viral Diseases" at Wuhan University will hole its tenth biennial meeting at Wuhan, on July 29–31, 2016. The Organizing Committee for the conference wishes to make the meeting an international one, inviting many famous foreign scientists who share common interests in the field. The official languages to be used in the conference will be Chinese and English.

Recently Professor Xiong Zhenming told me that you were interested in the symposium and the Organizing Committee would like you to attend the meeting to give a paper introducing your recent findings on any subjects related to viral diseases.

Your expenses in connection with attending the meeting, including travel from and to New York transportation, lodging and board in Wuhan, will be paid by the Organizing Committee.

Please advise me of your availability and provide me with your passport number, so that we may send you the visa application form.

Upon receiving your affirmative answer, we will send you a formal invitation and further information.

Yours sincerely,

Xiang Tianming

Chairman, CVD X

5. 邀请参加校庆（An invitation to attend a college celebration）

亲爱的 ××× 博士：

为了庆祝 ×× 医学院建校40周年，校友会决定举行"10 月 20 日庆祝会"。

我们热诚邀请您前来参加庆祝会。庆祝会将在外宾楼餐厅举行，时间定为10 月 19 日，上午 10 点 30 分开始，下午 2 点 30 分结束。

当日活动安排如下：

（1）早晨10 点 30 分至中午 12 点，校友会主席 ××× 致欢迎辞，副院长 ××× 将报告我院在教育方面取得的新成就。

（2）中午 12 点至下午 1 点 30 分，午饭。餐厅将为大家提供各式各样的地方风味菜肴。

（3）下午 1 点 30 分至 2 点 30 分，在学校花园举行音乐茶话会。所有的客人欢聚一堂，还可以欣赏一些中国音乐。届时将为大家提供水果、饮料。

请尽快告诉我您能否出席庆祝会。我们期待着您的肯定回答。

×× 医学院校友会

您的真诚的

×××

Sept. 20, 2016

Dr. ...

President & Professor

University of Cleveland

Cleveland, Ohio 31289

Dear Dr. ...,

To mark the 40th anniversary of the establishment of ... Medical College, the Alumni Association of ... Medical college has arranged to sponsor an "October 20th Celebration".

You are cordially invited to join us in the celebration of this occasion. The program will be held in the Dining Hall of Foreign Guest House, Saturday, October 19th from 10:30 a.m. to 2:30 p.m.

The plan for the day is as follows:

(1) 10:30—12:00 a.m., Mr. ..., Chairman of the Alumni Association, will give the welcoming address. Mr. ..., Vice President of our College, will speak on new achievements in education of our College.

(2) 12:00—1:30 p.m. Luncheon, Dining Hall. Various local-style dishes will be served.

(3) 1:30—2:30 p.m. Music and Talk in the Campus Garden. All guests will have a chance to meet each other and enjoy some Chinese music. Fruit and drinks will be served in the garden.

Please let us know as soon as possible if you can attend this celebration. We look forward to your positive reply.

Sincerely yours,

(Signature)

...

Alumni Association

... Medical College

6. 邀请参加落成典礼（An invitation to attend a dedication of project）

亲爱的 ××× 博士：

　　我十分荣幸地邀请您于 2016 年 8 月 27 日（周六）来参加我院新口腔医院的落成典礼。

　　典礼将由 ×× 医学院院领导和新口腔医院院长主持。

　　我渴望您能带来我们姐妹学校得克萨斯大学口腔学院的问候。您可以讲述两校建立的关系和互派人员工作；可以评论贵校在发展和促进与 ×× 医学院的合作和友好关系方面所发挥的作用；也可以评述任何有关口腔教育方面的国际交流成果，您的致辞可用 3~4 分钟。

　　我们为您在承德友谊宾馆预订了房间。您的日程一经确定，请即告诉我详情，以便安排人到机场迎接。为使您的旅游愉快，您对我们的安排还有任何特殊要求，亦请告知，当尽力照办。

您的真诚的

××× 博士

June 30, 2016

Dr. …

Dean

College of Allied Health Sciences

Thomas Jefferson University

Philadelphia, PA19307

Dear Dr. …,

　　It is indeed my pleasure to invite you to participate in the Dedication Ceremony of our new University Dental Hospital on

Saturday, August 27, 2016.

The Dedication will be conducted primarily by ... Medical College's Regents and the President of the New University Dental Hospital.

I would like very much for you to bring a brief greeting from our sister school, the Dental Branch of the University of Texas. You could comment on the initiation of our relationship and the faculty exchange programs we have enjoyed. You also could comment about your college's role in developing cooperation and promoting friendship with ... Medical College. Any comments about the benefits of international relations in dental education would be appropriated. Your brief comments should extend for three to four minutes.

We have made tentative hotel reservations for you at the Chengde Friendship Hotel. As soon as your itinerary is confirmed, please let me know the details so that we can make arrangements for you to be met at the airport. If there is anything we can do to make your trip more pleasant, or if there are any special arrangements you would like us to make while you are in Chengde, please do not hesitate to let me know.

Sincerely yours,

(Signature)

..., M.D.

7. 邀请参加宴会（An invitation to attend a banquet）

亲爱的×××博士：

　　×××博士已通知我，您将于8月来参加我院新口腔医院的落成典礼，我感到十分高兴。

　　落成典礼结束后，我院将于8月27日晚6点30分在友谊俱乐部设晚宴酬宾。

如您能出席晚宴,我们将倍感荣幸。请尽快告诉我您能否出席,以便再做出必要安排。典礼会上见,届时再确认所做的安排。

您的真诚的

× × ×

July 11, 2016

Dr. ...

Dean

College of Allied Health Sciences

Thomas Jefferson University

Philadelphia, PA 19107

Dear Dr. ...,

Dr. ... has indicated to me that you will attend the Dedication Ceremony of our new Dental Hospital in August. I am very pleased to hear that you will attend.

Following the Dedication Ceremony, our College will sponsor a dinner at the Friendship Club on Saturday, August 27, at 6:30 p.m.

We would be honored to have you as our guest at the dinner. Please notify me as soon as possible whether or not you will be able to attend so that I can make the necessary arrangements. We will see you at the Dedication Ceremony, and confirm our arrangements.

Sincerely yours,

(Signature)

...

8. 邀请参加授衔仪式（An invitation to commencement）

亲爱的 ××× 博士：

　　如您所知，××× 博士将于 2017 年 6 月 9 日接受 ×× 医学院授予的名誉博士称号。他将于 6 月 7 日抵达承德，6 月 11 日离开。

　　我希望您能有暇作为我的客人来参加授予仪式。我院将为您提供国际旅费，并承担您在承德期间的费用。

　　盼望见到您。

您的真诚的

××× 博士

March 8th, 2017

Dr. ...

Dean and Vice President

School of Medicine

The Univ. of Parramatta

Westmead, NSW 2145

Dear Dr. ...,

　　As you know, Dr. ... will receive an honorary doctor degree from ... Medical College on June 9, 2017. He is scheduled to arrive in Chengde on June 7 and leave on June 11.

　　I hope that you will be free to join us as my guest, when we honor him in Chengde. The College will reimburse you for your air travel to and from China, and cover your expenses in Chengde as well.

　　Looking forward to seeing you.

Sincerely,

(Signature)

..., M.D.

9. 邀请讲学（An invitation to deliver lectures）

亲爱的 ××× 博士：

　　我代表 ×× 医学院对您在过去 3 年间为发展我们的医学教育工作所做的努力表示感谢。我们还特别对贵系的 ××× 教授表示感谢，他为学生讲解了十分有意义的课程。毒理学和致畸学是中国学者急需了解的两门课程。

　　如果您能再来中国与专业人员举行几次讨论会我们将十分高兴。我希望您能抽暇来访，并对您 2014 年访问之后我们所做的工作进行评价。

　　请告诉我您成行的可能性，并请告知您和夫人的护照号码，以便寄上签证申请表。

　　致以良好的问候。

　　　　　　　　　　　　　　　　　　　　　您的真诚的

　　　　　　　　　　　　　　　　　　　　　　×××

Sept. 3, 2016

..., M.D.

Chairman & Professor

Dept. of Pharmacology & Toxicology

University of Louisville

Louisville, KY 40292

Dear Dr. ...,

On behalf of ... Medical College I would like to express our great appreciation of your efforts to enhance our medical education over the last three years. We are especially grateful to Prof. ... of your department for coming here to teach courses which were of great benefit to our medical students. Toxicology and Teratology are two subjects which our Chinese professionals need desperately to understand.

We would be happy to have you return and give a couple of seminars for our faculty. I hope you can take time off to visit us and to evaluate our progress since your last visit in 2014.

Please advise me about your availability, and provide me with your and your wife's passport numbers, so that we may send you the visa application form.

With best regards,

Sincerely yours,

(Signature)

…

*　　　*　　　*

亲爱的×××博士：

我十分荣幸地邀请您来我院讲学。

您的《代谢性骨病的镁代谢》一书一经出版就引起了中国同行们的极大兴趣。此外，您随即发表的有关这一方面的出版物及所做的讲座已使您声名大振。我们非常欢迎您来阐述这一方面的最新观点并愿和您讨论。因此，如您能来我院进行系列讲座，我们将十分荣幸。

您的旅费和住宿费将由我院负责。我们还将陪您到承德附近的几个风景区去旅游。

请告诉我们您是否能来以及来的时间。欢迎您与我们共同讨论您的讲课计划。

顺致最美好的祝愿。

您的真诚的

×××博士

June 8, 2016

Prof. ...
Dept. of System Science
Univ. of New York
New York, N. Y. 10056

Dear Prof. ...,

I am very pleased to have the honor of inviting you for an academic tour of our College.

As soon as your book "The Magnesium Metabolism of Metabolic Bone Disorders" came of the press, it kindled a lot of interest in the minds of many Chinese experts in this field. Moreover, your subsequent publications and lectures on the subject have won you credit and popularity. We would very much welcome an opportunity to hear your latest views and to discuss them further with you. Therefore, we would consider it a great honor if you could come to our College to give this series of talks.

Your travel and hotel expenses will be paid by our College. We will also provide a tour to some scenic spots around Chengde.

Please let us know if you are able to come, and when you might do so. You are also welcome to discuss your lecture program with us.

With best wishes,

Sincerely yours,
(Signature)
..., M.D.

10. 邀请来华工作（An invitation to work in China）

亲爱的 ×××博士：

我十分荣幸地聘请您为 ×× 医学院客座教授，从 2017 年

2月1日至2018年1月31日来我院工作。您将在我院解剖教研室与教师们一道工作，并承担五年制医学生解剖课的某些章节的教学工作。

尽管学院的工作场所有限，但××博士已在科里为您做了妥善的准备，他将安排您在我院外宾宿舍住宿，您的每月工资为5 000元人民币。

除与××博士共事外，我们也乐意安排您去其他教研室参与工作，以便您适应我们的教学计划和教学方法。既然您对病理生理学很感兴趣，如您愿意，我们将为您在那个教研室安排一定的工作时间。

随信附上一封正式邀请信，您可凭它到中国使馆办理签证。您还有何问题或建议请写信告知。

顺致良好祝愿。

您的真诚的

×××博士

April 30, 2016

…, M.D.

Dept. of Anatomy

School of Medicine

Univ. of Texas

Houston, Texas 77225

Dear Dr. …,

It is my pleasure to offer you a visiting professorship at … Medical College beginning Feb. 1, 2017 and ending Jan. 31, 2018. Your appointment would entail working with faculty in the Department of Anatomy of our College and deliver some chapters of Anatomy Textbook to our five-year medical students.

Although space is at a premium at the institute, Dr. ... will make provisions for you to work in his department. He also will make arrangements for you to have a room in the Foreign Guest House of our College. The monthly salary associated with this position is RMB 5,000 yuan.

In addition to working with Dr. ..., we would be most happy to have you work in other departments in our College and to orientate you to our curriculum and methods of teaching. Since you have a particular interest in pathophysiology, we will arrange for you to spend time in that department, if you wish.

Accompanying this letter, please find an official invitation letter, with which you can apply for entry visa from the Chinese Embassy. Should you have any questions or comments, please do not hesitate to let me know.

With best regards,

Sincerely yours,
(Signature)
..., M.D.

*　　　*　　　*

亲爱的 ×××博士：

我非常高兴地获悉，您愿采取某种方式为祖国的发展与实现现代化做出贡献。您甘愿奉献的精神给我留下了深刻的印象。我们对愿为祖国做出贡献的所有人士表示欢迎。

从来信得知您愿做口腔医生工作并打算举办一些讲座。这一想法令人激动，必将对我们的医学教育大有裨益。希望您能将讲座的题目提供给我们。了解了您的想法之后，我们可以为您的来访做出具体安排。

请早日赐复。

您的真诚的
××× 博士

August 3rd, 2016

..., D. D. S.
955 Union Street
San Francisco
California 94133

Dear Dr, ...,

I am very pleased to know that you want to contribute in some way to our ancestral homeland's development and to aid in the modernization of our country. Your willingness to help us has left a lasting impression on me. We welcome all persons who wish to give something back to the land of their ancestors.

From your letter we know you wish offer your services as a dentist and deliver some lectures as well. The idea is an exciting one and would certainly be of assistance to our medical education. I hope that you will provide us with a list of topics on which you would like to lecture. We need to have your ideas so that we can make concrete arrangements for your visit.

Please let us hear from you soon.

Sincerely yours,
(Signature)
..., M.D.

11. 邀请参加科研工作（An invitation to join in research work）

亲爱的 ×××博士：

兹致函邀请您参加流行病学或公共卫生学的研究工作。

我希望您能接受邀请。我们将争取资金，以承担您在承德两周期间的费用。我们准备为您提供香港至承德的往返旅费和在承德的食宿。

您的真诚的

×××博士

Nov. 14, 2016

…, M.D.

Prof. of Microbiology

Dept of Microbiology

Univ. of Hong Kong

Dear Dr. …,

Please accept this letter as an invitation to participate in research activities in the field of epidemiology or public health.

I hope you will be able to accept our invitation. We will make funds available to cover the costs of your two-week stay in Chengde. We are prepared to finance your travel expenses from and to Hong Kong as well as provide our accommodations in Chengde.

Sincerely yours,

(Signature)

…, M.D.

第二节　答复邀请信
（Replies to Invitation）

在接到对方邀请信后，不管接受与否，必须及时答复，否则有失礼貌。这类复信要写得热情、简洁。这类信应包括以下几个方面的内容。

（1）首先感谢对方的邀请。

（2）愉快接受对方的邀请。如不能接受，首先感谢对方的盛情邀请，并对不能应邀表示遗憾；然后简单陈述不能应邀的原因；同时可表示以后能赴邀的时间。最后可写希望以后能有机会见面，或向邀请人致以问候。

（3）表示期待如期赴约的心情。

1. 接受邀请（Replies to Invitation）

亲爱的×××博士：

感谢您来信确认邀请我们访问路易斯威尔，对此我们感到十分荣幸。我已写信给我院×××院长，以确定我们出访的适当时间。

我的夫人是一位教育工作者，她必须向单位请假。出访日期一经确定，她就去请假。

十分感谢您为此事帮忙，再次感谢您的盛情邀请。

您的真诚的

×××

Oct. 21, 2016

..., Ph. D.
Chairman & Professor
Department of Physiology
School of Medicine
University of Louisville
Louisville, Kentucky 40292

Dear Dr. ...,

　　Thank you for your letter confirming our invitation to visit Louisville. I am honoured by your invitation. I have written to Dr. ..., President of our college, requesting confirmation of the appropriate dates for our visit.

　　Since my wife is an educator, she, too, must receive permission for a leave of absence from her institution. She will apply for her leave as soon as the dates of our visit are confirmed.

　　We are grateful for your help in this matter, and again express our appreciation for your gracious invitation.

Sincerely,
(Signature)
...

2. 接受邀请去做研究工作（Acceptance of an invitation to do research）

亲爱的 ××× 博士：

　　感谢您在 2017 年 11 月 14 日的来信。我十分荣幸地接受您的邀请，去参观贵系并进行为期两个月的有关流行病和公共卫生的研究工作。我愉快地接受邀请并盼望着访问香港。

　　关于我研究的内容，我同意您的建议，并将尽快把具体计划寄上。

　　再次感谢您盛情邀请并希望此次出访对双方都有裨益。

　　致以良好的祝愿。

您的真诚的

×××

Dec. 4, 2017

Dr. ...

Professor of Microbiology

Head of Department

University of Hong Kong

Queen Mary Hospital

Hong Kong

Dear Dr. ...,

　　Thank you very much for your letter of November 14, 2017. I am greatly honoured to have your invitation to visit your department for two months to carry out research activities in the field of epidemiology and public health. I accept, with pleasure, and look forward to visiting Hong Kong.

　　Regarding the contents of my research, I agree to your proposal, and I will send you a detailed outline as soon as possible.

　　Again, thank you very much for your kind invitation. I hope that the visit will be mutually beneficial.

　　With best regards,

Sincerely yours,

(Signature)

..., M.D.

3. 接受邀请去讲学(Acceptance of an invitation to give lectures)

亲爱的 ×××博士：

感谢您 2016 年 1 月 22 日的来信。我乐于接受您的邀请，到贵校讲授头颈部解剖学。

您的来信我已呈×××院长阅示，您来我校访问时曾会见过他。×××院长欣然同意我暂时离校，于 6 月初到贵校任教。

我正忙于安排日程并组织其他与头颈部解剖有关的教材。一旦材料完成，我就寄给您，以便您着手准备工作。

再次感谢您的邀请，盼望 6 月初在费城晤面。

您的真诚的

×××博士

May 31, 2016

…, Ph. D.

Dean

Dental Department

University of Penn

Philadelphia, PA 19104

Dear Dr. …,

Thank you for your letter of January 22, 2016. I am delighted to receive your invitation to teach "Head & Neck" anatomy in your medical school and eagerly accept.

I have presented your letter to our President, Dr. …, who you met while visiting our College. He has graciously granted me permission for the temporary leave needed to teach in your College beginning in June.

I am in the process of organizing a schedule and other relevant information regarding the "Head & Neck" anatomy class. As soon as the information is completed, I will send it to you so that you can initiate any necessary preparatory work.

Thank you again for your invitation. I am looking forward to seeing you in early June in Philadelphia.

Sincerely yours,
(Signature)
…, M.D.

＊　　　＊　　　＊

亲爱的×××博士：

首先，我想您回国旅程一定安全、轻松而顺利。您读到这封信时，想必已体轻神怡、恢复到"正常"状态了。

我十分乐于接受您的邀请，明年7月到明尼苏达大学去讲学。我已安排好访问贵校的计划，7月17日到达，一直待到7月20日。目前我的计划是一天讲学，二天旅游，初步考虑参观明尼阿波利斯附近的几个名胜。

请协助我与负责此次讲座的人员联系上，希望讲学的题目合适，能使您和同事们感兴趣。

很高兴得知您明年11月份将访问承德，盼望届时能为您效劳。

致以良好的祝愿。

您的真诚的
×××

June 29, 2016

..., M.D.

Professor of Pediatrics

Chairman

Dept. of Cardiology

University of Minnesota

Minneapolis, Minnesota 55455

Dear Dr. ...,

First, may I say that I hope your journey home was safe, relaxing and uneventful. By the time you read my letter, hopefully you will have had a chance to relax and adjust to being back in a "normal" situation.

I am happy to accept your invitation to deliver lectures next July at University of Minnesota. I have completed the arrangements for my visit to your University. I will be arriving on July 17 and will be there through July 20. My present plan is for a one–day lecture, followed by two days of traveling primarily to visit some ancient places near Minneapolis.

Please put me in contact with the persons who will be specifically involved with my lectures. I hope that the subjects are appropriate and are of interest to you and your staff.

It is a pleasure to learn of your plans to visit Chengde next November. I look forward to the opportunity to be of service to you upon your arrival.

With best wishes,

Sincerely yours,

(Signature)

...

4. 推迟赴邀日期（Postponing）

亲爱的 ××× 博士：

　　××× 博士近期刚从东卡罗林纳大学访问归来,带来了您给我的友好邀请,对此我十分感激,但这次我不得不将访问日程推迟至 2016 年底或 2017 年初。

　　目前,我在本院有许多科研与教学任务,另外在其他医学院的科研与教学工作也十分繁忙,实难脱身。

　　再一次感谢您的盛情邀请,并希望今后就有关学术交流问题相互交换意见。

您的真诚的
××× 博士

July 18, 2015

..., Ph. D.
Professor of Pathophysiology
School of Medicine
East Carolina University
Greenville, North Carolina 27834

Dear Dr. ...,

　　Dr. ... recently returned from a visit to East Carolina University and brought me your very kind invitation to visit your institution. I am most appreciative, but at this time I must defer acceptance until sometime late in 2016 or early in 2017.

　　At the present time I have a series of commitments to research and teaching in the College as well as a very active research and teaching schedule in other medical Colleges.

　　Once again I thank you for your invitation and hope that we may communicate with regard to an academic exchange at a later time.

Sincerely yours,
(Signature)
…, M.D.

* * *

亲爱的×××博士：

收到您 2016 年 3 月 3 日的来信,十分高兴。由于今天刚收到,迟复为歉。能够到贵中心讲学,感到十分荣幸。

我非常愿意赴约,但学院还有许多后勤问题亟待解决,因此现在还不能给您一个肯定的答复。我们期待着×××博士的 10 月来访,待他来时我可能与他商谈此事。您愿为我和我的夫人承担在密苏里的费用,感人至深。我也希望能解决一些与我的访问有关的问题。我愿审慎考虑讲学的内容,以便能对贵所人员有所裨益。

我清楚地记得您的来访,并十分想念您。我的确感到我现在已有很多美国朋友,当然也包括您在内。尽管我们远隔千里,但我们息息相通。

待我做出肯定的答复并确定了感兴趣的讲学题目后即行奉告。

您的真诚的
×××博士

April 4, 2016

..., M.D.
Department of Radiology
Boone Hospital Center
Calumbia, Missouri 65201

Dear Dr. ...,

I was delighted to receive your letter of March 3, 2016. It arrived only today and thus delay my response, I am flattered by your invitation to deliver a lecture in your center.

I would like very much to do so, but there are a number of logistic problems and it is not possible at this moment for me to give you a firm answer. We anticipate a visit from Dr. ... in October and perhaps when he comes I will be able to discuss this with him. You are very kind to offer to cover the expenses for me and my wife in Missouri. I hope to be able to work out some of the problems associated with my visiting you and your college. Also, I want to think seriously about what I might be able to present which would be useful to individuals associated with your institution.

I remember your visit so well and I miss you. I truly feel that I now have a number of friends, you included, of course, in America and though we are separated by several thousand miles, we are united in other ways.

I shall let you know when I can make a firm commitment and what topics of interest I might cover.

Sincerely yours,
(Signature)
..., M.D.

5. 接受邀请但要求缩短访问时间（Acceptance of an invitation but requesting a shorter stay）

亲爱的 ××× 博士：

今天刚收到您的邀请信。我急于告诉您的是，能在 2016 年 10 月 20 日访问休斯顿我感到十分高兴。我非常乐于向您和您的同事们介绍 ×× 医学院的最新研究情况以及把这些成果结合到您的研究计划中去。

由于在国内有系列讲座要讲，我不能在您可爱的国家停留太长时间，尽管我希望那样。我的飞行计划确定后，就立即告诉您最新消息。我们计划 10 月 17 日离开中国，以确保 20 日（周一）到达休斯顿，在贵院休息，并为会议做准备。

怀着崇敬的心情，盼望着 10 月份见到您。

我对您和您的家人致以良好的祝愿。

您的真诚的

××× 博士

Sept. 2, 2016

…, Ph. D.

Professor of Ophthalmology

Baylor College of Medicine

Houston, TX 77030

Dear Prof. …,

Your invitation arrived just today, and I hasten to reply that I will be most pleased to be in Houston on October 20, 2016. It will give me great pleasure to present to you and your colleagues some of the latest studies here at … Medical College and how they might be incorporated into your study curriculum.

Due to the pressures of my seminar series here, I will be unable to spend as much time in your lovely country as I would wish. I will notify you as soon as my flight plans are definite. We plan to depart from China on October 17 to ensure our arrival in Houston on Monday, the 20th and to be rested for our meeting at your university.

With much respect and looking forward to seeing you in October. My very best wishes to your family.

Sincerely yours,

(Signature)

…, M.D.

6. 婉辞邀请（Declining an invitation）

亲爱的×××博士：

感谢您5月31日来信盛情邀请我到伦敦访问和讲学。

然而，无论是今年秋天还是明年秋天都有问题。今年8月份，我们将在国内进行为期1个月的旅行，这意味着我今年不能离开我的岗位。明年秋天，我已确定到意大利米兰出席国际肉瘤会议，并做报告。其后，我还没做出其他安排。请相信，对您邀请我到贵国访问，我感到十分荣幸。

也许将来某个时候，若时间和健康状况允许，我们可再商谈此事。再次感谢您友好的邀请，此次未能成行，至感歉疚。

您的真诚的

×××博士

June 23, 2016

..., M.D.
Chairman
Dept. of Physiology
King's College
Strand, London
England

Dear Dr. ...,

Thank you very much for your letter of May 31, 2016 and your gracious invitation to visit and lecture in London.

However, to make the trip this fall or next presents a problem. This August, we will be gone on a month-long trip within China which means that I cannot absent myself from my duties at Medical College any time this year. Next fall, I have already committed myself to delivering a paper at the International Sarcoidosis Meeting in Milan, Italy. Beyond that I hesitate to make any commitment. Believe me, I am flattered and honored that you wish me to come to your city.

Perhaps at some future time, if events and health permit we might discuss this matter again. Again thank you very much for your kind offer, and I apologize I am unable to accept.

Sincerely yours,
(Signature)
..., M.D.

第三节 感谢信(Appreciation)

感谢信是为感谢对方的关心、支持、帮助或馈赠而写的信。

在应邀赴宴、收到礼品或得到别人帮助之后，及时写一封感谢信是非常必要的。这是一个惯例，也是一种礼貌。感谢信的语言要恳切，感情要真挚，通常还应提及对方的帮助怎么重要，招待的如何周到等。

感谢信一般是一个较大的段落，但分成几个小段也可以。其内容通常包括以下 3 个方面：

（1）对对方提供的帮助、给予的接待或赠送的礼品表示感谢。

（2）简单说明对方提供的帮助所起的作用或赠送礼品的将来用途。

（3）再次感谢或问候对方。

1. 感谢学术合作（Appreciation for academic cooperation）

亲爱的 ××× 博士：

这是一封迟复的感谢信，感谢您为安排我去哈佛医学院实验室参观所做的一切。对您的热情款待，我实在感激不尽，简直难以用语言表达。

这次访问中，我们的会谈卓有成效。特别是您对 ×× 医学院护理教育的支持使人难以忘怀。您对护理学学士教育的支持将大大加速护理项目的发展。我确信，这对两校之间的理解与进一步合作至关重要。如还有什么事情要我来做，即请告知，当竭尽全力。

再次感谢您的盛情和您的慷慨。

您的真诚的

×××

June 17, 2017

…, M.D.

Harvard Medical School

Boston Massachusetts 02115

Dear Dr. …,

This is a long overdue letter to thank you for arranging my visit to the research laboratories at Harvard Medical School. I just want you to know how overwhelmed I am by your kind hospitality. I enjoyed my visit more than I can put into words.

We had some very productive discussions during this trip. I was particularly impressed by your support of nursing education at … Medical College. Your support of baccalaureate education in nursing will do much to advance the cause of nursing projects, but we believe they are very important to the understanding and further collaboration between our two institutions. If there is anything I can do for you, please don't hesitate to ask.

Again, thank you for everything … your kindness and your generosity.

Sincerely yours,

(Signature)

…, M.D.

2. 感谢款待并提出合作建议（Appreciation for hospitality and put forward the cooperation）

亲爱的×××博士：

我相信没有更恰当的词语可用来表达对您的感激之情了，万分感谢您为我在贵国度过的充实而令人激动的两个月所做的一切。您的热情招待，感人至深。那次访问和您的友谊，我将永志不忘。

　　我怀着万分感激的心情清楚地记得，您为我做出了细致而周密的安排；在休斯顿机场接我，带我在休斯顿和佛罗里达观光。更为荣幸的是见到了您那可亲可敬的家人。您的家宴是地道的西方风味，真是妙不可言。最重要的是，您的热情款待和您的友谊使我记忆犹新。贵校校长×××博士和我的朋友们为我举行的宴会，所赠礼品以及聘任我为贵校课座教授都特别值得感谢。

　　我在休斯顿及贵国其他城市访问期间，有许许多多令人难忘的时光，但最令人难忘的是能到贵校参观访问。贵校的设备、工作质量都给我留下了深刻的印象。教师们那充满激情的献身精神令人钦佩。我希望这次访问将进一步增进××医学院与休斯顿社区大学间的相互交流和进一步合作。我以个人的名义，并代表××医学院对探讨这种合作的可能性表示极大的关注，并期待着贵校给予有力的支持。

　　再一次对您在我访美期间所给予的热情接待和盛情款待表示诚挚谢意。

您的真诚的
×××博士

July 18, 2016

…, M.D.
Prof. & Chairman
Houston Community College
Houston, Texas 77270

Dear Professor …,

　　I don't believe there are appropriate words to adequately thank you for all that you did for me during my fulfilled, exciting two-month swing through the States. Your hospitality was just superb and I will cherish that visit and your friendship forever.

I remember vividly and with great appreciation all the nice arrangements you made for me, meeting us at Houston Airport, sightseeing with us in Houston and Florida. We were very honored, too, to be your house guests and enjoyed meeting the lovely and talented members of your family. The real western-style dinner at your home was great. Most of all, the warm hospitality and your great friendship will remain fresh in my memory. The banquet hosted by Dr. ..., President of your University, and my friends (which you gave in my honour), the gift, and my Visiting Professor appointment are especially appreciated.

There were many highlights of my visit to Houston and your country, but nothing was more appreciated than the opportunity to visit your university. I was very impressed with the facilities and the quality of work being done. The obvious enthusiasm and dedication of your faculty member are heartwarming. I hope this visit will promote further interaction and collaboration between the ... Medical College and Houston Community College. I personally, and as a representative of ... Medical College, am very interested in exploring this possibility and anticipate the concept being strongly supported by your University.

Once again, I want to express my gratitude for the very warm reception, and wonderful hospitality which was extended to me during my visit.

Sincerely yours,
(Signature)
..., M.D.

3. 感谢状（Certificate of appreciation）

感　谢　状

　　×××女士于2017年9月22日至12月20日访问了承德。应××医学院邀请，×××女士为护理界举办了生动的讲座。她的讲座深受欢迎，获得成功，对承德护理界十分有益。我十分荣幸地代表××医学院对×××女士为护理科学和××医学院与托马斯·杰佛逊大学之间的友谊所做的有益贡献表示感谢。

××医学院院长

×××

2017年12月20日

CERTIFICATE OF APPRECIATION

　　Ms. … has visited Chengde from September 22 to December 20, 2017. Mr. … has given interesting lectures to the nurses at the invitation of … Medical College. Her lectures are welcome, very successful and very helpful to the nursing field in Chengde. I have the pleasure to thank her on behalf of … Medical College for her valuable contribution to the cause of nursing science and to the friendship between … Medical College and Thomas Jefferson University.

…, M.D.

President

… Medical College

The People's Republic of China

December 20, 2017

4. 感谢被聘任为客座教授（Appreciation for a visiting professorship）

亲爱的×××博士：

在最近访问贵院期间，我受到您和口腔学院全体教师和学生们的热情招待，对此我表示衷心感谢。对贵院授予我口腔科学客座教授称号尤感荣幸，这种殊荣我将永远引以自豪。

简言之，我们这次得克萨斯之行是令人愉快，卓有成效而富有意义的，我们也受到其他医学院校的热情招待，进行了有意义的讲学并和美国同行商谈。

我现在已回到承德，正忙于处理我不在时积攒起来的工作。看来还得需要一段时间，我才能翻阅完办公桌上的材料，但我还是想花些时间来表达对您的感谢之情。

我们希望继续发展两校之间的关系并同您保持持久的友谊。

盼望着在承德或休斯顿再次见面。

您的真诚的

×××

April 28, 2016

Dean …, D. D. S.

Dental Branch

The University of Texas

Houston, Texas 77225

Dear Dr. …,

Please accept my sincerest appreciation for the hospitality extended by you, the faculty, and student body of the Dental School on my recent visit to your prestigious university. Needless to say, I am greatly honored by my appointment as Visiting Professor of Stomatology to your University. It is a tribute I will always be proud of.

In short, our trip to the Texas was enjoyable, productive and meaningful. We were well received by the other medical schools and enjoyed presenting lectures and consulting with them.

Now I am back in Chengde trying to catch up on all of the work which piled up while I was gone. It will be sometime before I can see over the paper on my desk, but, I did want to take a few minutes to express to you my sincere thanks for everything you did for me.

We look forward to a growing relationship between our two institutions and a lasting friendship with you.

We hope to see you again soon both here in Chengde and in Houston.

Sincerely,

(Signature)

…

5. 感谢关照(Appreciation for being taken good care of)

亲爱的 ××× 教授：

    我的同事,电子显微镜实验室主任技师 ××× 先生,在贵系访问期间受到热烈欢迎,对此谨向您表示衷心感谢。我对您和您的同事们给予他热诚的帮助和指导也表示诚挚谢意。正是由于您不懈地帮助,××× 先生才在我们共同感兴趣的实验性碘缺乏羊克汀病研究方面获得卓有成效的训练。

    盼望着香港大学与 ×× 医学院进一步加强医学教育与科学研究的合作。

顺致春节问候。

您的真诚的

×××博士

Jan. 28, 2017

Prof. ...

Dept. of Pathophysiology

Queen Mary Hospital

Univ. of Hong Kong

Dear Professor ...,

I wish to extend my deepest appreciation to you for welcoming my colleague Mr. ..., chief technician of our electromicroscopy laboratory while he was an observer in your department. I also thank you for the valuable help and guidance rendered to him by you and your staff. It is entirely through your unceasing effort that Mr. ... obtained excellent laboratory training in experimental iodine deficiency lamb cretinism research, an area of common interest.

Looking forward to closer collaboration in medical education and research between the University of Hong Kong and ... Medical College.

With traditional lunar calender new year greetings.

Sincerely yours,

(Signature)

..., M.D.

6. 感谢被接见（Appreciation for being met）

亲爱的 ×××博士：

有幸于 2017 年 11 月 21 日周三晚上在费城见到您，十分高兴。您在百忙之中接见我，我十分感激。您为我抵美访问和在费城做短暂停留精心安排，这一切都使我感激不尽。尽管时间匆匆，但感到十分愉快。

如您再来访问承德，作我的客人，我将格外高兴。

致以良好的个人问候。

您的真诚的

×××

Nov. 26, 2017

…, D. D. S.

2008 Walnut Street

Philadelphia, PA 19103

Dear Dr. …,

It was a pleasure for me to meet with you in Philadelphia on Wednesday evening, November 21, 2017. I am particularly grateful to you for having taken time out of your busy schedule to meet me and I do want to thank you for all you did to assure that my arrival in the States and my short stay in Philadelphia was well–managed and comfortable. Although the time spent was short I enjoyed it enormously.

Should you visit Chengde again, I will be pleased to have you visit me.

With best personal regards,

Sincerely yours,

(Signature)

…, M.D.

7. 感谢被允许参观一个科室(Appreciation for being allowed to visit a department)

亲爱的霍克斯教授：

首先非常感谢您允许我参观您的科室并观摩心脏直视手术,我对此非常感兴趣。

您能否费心寄给我一篇您文章的复印稿(篇名为心脏直视手术,2016 年发表于《外科》杂志,第 4 卷,第 26 期)?

您的忠诚的

Hussain Ismail(医生)

Department of Cardiology.

Guy's Hospital

London SEI

21 December 2017

Professor C Hocks

Department of Cardiology

St Thomas' Hospital

London SEI

Dear Professor Hocks,

Thank you so much for allowing me to visit your department and to watch some open-heart surgery being performed. It was interesting to me.

I wonder if you would be so kind as to send me a copy of your reprint: Hocks, C.: Open–heart surgery, *Surgery* 26, 4, 2016?

Yours sincerely

Hussain Ismail (Dr.)

8. 感谢教授英语(Appreciation for an English course)

亲爱的×××博士:

我真不知用多少词汇才能表达我对您所给予的帮助的感激之情。

不用说,×××博士来我院访问是我院极大的荣幸。×××博士在我院访问了3个月并出色地讲授了英语课程。她严谨治学,给我们留下了深刻印象。她的辛勤劳动得到了回报。同学们对她那精湛的教学技术以及热爱同学的真挚感情都给予了高度评价。我相信,她此次讲学是愉快的、有成效的,而且是有意义的,并相信她的科学贡献将促进我院医学教育的发展和教学水平的提高。

我谨代表××医学院向×××博士表示衷心感谢,感谢她为发展医学教育以及得克萨斯大学医学院和××医学院之间的友谊做出的贡献。

致以良好的问候。

您的真诚的

×××博士

May 25, 2017

Dr. ...
Dean
The University of Texas
Medical School at Houston
Houston, Texas 77225

Dear Dr. ...,

I don't believe there are enough words to adequately thank you for the great support you have extended to us.

Needless to say, we are greatly honored to have Dr. ... visit our College. Dr. ... spent three months at our College and she delivered an excellent English course. We were impressed by her scholarly performances. Her hard work has been fully rewarded. Her students hold her in great esteem not only for her consummate teaching skill, but also for her great love for the students. Her lecture trip has been, I am sure, enjoyable, productive and meaningful. I believe that her scientific contribution will help us promote medical education and raise our teaching standards.

I wish to thank her on behalf of ... Medical College for her valuable contribution to medical education and to friendship between ... Medical College and the Medical School of the University of Texas.

With our best regards,

Sincerely yours,
(Signature)
..., M.D.

9. 感谢赠送礼品（Appreciation for a gift）

亲爱的 ×××博士：

2016 年 12 月 13 日,贵院代表向 ××医学院正式赠送了纽约临床基金会的礼品。我们荣幸地收到了这尊自由女神像,它将是我们两校持久友谊的象征。我们还计划把它放在我院明年建成的新建筑物的显著位置展出,以便人人都能观赏它。

×院长和我对您向我们发出择时访问美国的友好邀请表示感谢。我们非常愿意前往,但不知 2017 年是否能实现。

再一次衷心感谢您赠送给我们珍贵的礼品,我们希望您不久再来访问。

致以良好的祝愿。

您的真诚的

×××博士

March 4, 2017

..., M.D.

Chairman

Board of Governors

The New York Clinic Foundation

New York, N. Y. 10043

Dear Dr. ...,

On December 13, 2016, representatives of your medical staff formally presented your gift from the New York Clinic Foundation to ... Medical College. The magnificent Statue of Liberty is gratefully received and will serve as a symbol of lasting friendship between our two institutions. We propose to exhibit the statue in a prominent location in our College addition, which will be completed next year, so that everyone can enjoy it.

Dr. ... and I appreciate your kind invitation to visit America sometime in the future. We would like very much to do so, but doubt that it will be possible to do so in 2017.

Once again, please accept our heartfelt appreciation for your treasured gift. We hope to have the pleasure of a visit from you again in the near future.

With best regards,

Sincerely yours,
(Signature)
..., M.D.

10. 感谢帮助（Appreciation for help）

亲爱的 ××× 博士：

我想告诉您，对贵院生化系 ××× 博士的来访，我们 ×× 医学院特别是生化教研室是何等高兴。

××× 博士的访问活动卓有成效，为我们提供了宝贵经验。他的讲座受到教师和同学们的欢迎。他曾检查了我们的教学计划，并参加了我们的许多会议，并对中国与美国的医学教育过程进行了认真评价和比较。××× 博士和我定期商谈医学教育，我感到他是一位才华横溢、聪明过人的观察家。我们为拥有他而感到高兴，并盼望着在他继续逗留期间为我院做出贡献。

请您相信，我们将努力使 ××× 博士的 ×× 医学院之行过的尽可能愉快而有价值。我期待着不断加强两校的合作纽带。××× 博士对贵院的评价很高，贵国的医学教育与科研也给我们留下了深刻印象。

致以良好的祝愿和新年问候。

您的真诚的
×××

Jan. 17, 2017

..., Ph. D.
Professor & Chairman
Dept. of Biochemistry
School of Medicine
Temple University
Philadelphia, PA 19102

Dear Dr. ...,

　　I wish to tell you how pleased the ... Medical College, particularly the department of biochemistry are with the visit of Dr. ..., a faculty member of the department of biochemistry of your university.

　　Dr. ... 's activities have been a most productive and valuable experience for us. His lectures are appreciated by our medical faculty and students. He has had an opportunity to view our educational programs and to participate in many of our faculty activities. He has attended many of our seminars as an observer. Dr. ... has been carefully evaluating and comparing the process of medical education in China with that of the U. S. A. He and I meet regularly to discuss medical education and I have found him to be a brilliant and astute observer. We enjoy having him in the department and look forward to his continued activities throughout the remainder of his stay.

　　You can be sure that we are doing everything possible to make Dr. ... 's stay at the ... Medical College as pleasant and profitable as possible. I look forward to developing strong ties between your university and ours. Dr. ... speaks highly of his university, and we are impressed with medical education and research in the United States.

　　My best regards and best wishes for the New Year,

Sincerely yours,
(Signature)
..., M.D.

11. 感谢款待（Appreciation for hospitality）

亲爱的 ×××博士：

　　请原谅我没能及时给您回信。我和我夫人于6月中旬结束了难忘的美国之行，就马上投入到学术和行政工作中去。

　　访问期间，承蒙您热情款待，对此我谨表示衷心感谢。访问的各个方面都进行的非常顺利，真令人愉快。贵院提供的食宿和员工给予的帮助也都相当出色，特别是教师们对我们的热情招待十分感人，促使我确信并乐于继续加强我们两校之间的友好纽带。

　　为了使我们的访问愉快，您付出了宝贵的时间和精力，对此我们特别表示诚挚的谢意。从到费城机场迎候我们到来，到陪同我们去参观尼亚加拉大瀑布和华盛顿特区，我们将永远怀念我们的美国之行以及我们共同度过的时光。

　　再次对这次难忘的费城之行向您们表示深切的谢意和由衷的感谢之情。

　　致以衷心的问候，并祝成功和愉快。

您的真诚的

×××博士

June 30, 2017

…, Ph. D.

Professor & Chairman

Dept. Of Biochemistry

Hahnemann University

Philadelphia, PA 19102

Dear Dr. …,

　　Please excuse my delay for not writing to you earlier. My wife and I arrived home from our wonderful trip to America in mid-June, but I was immediately overwhelmed with academic and administrative tasks.

I wish to express to you our deepest appreciation for the warm hospitality you extended to us during our visit. Every aspect of the visit went smoothly and was an exciting experience. The accommodations and assistance provided by the staff of your university were excellent. The warmth and friendship offered to me by the faculty was wonderful and reinforces my conviction and desire to continue to develop stronger ties between our two medical colleges.

We are particularly grateful for all the time and effort you took to make our stay so enjoyable. From meeting us at the Philadelphia Airport to accompanying us on our trip to the Niagara Falls and the visit to Washington D. C., we will cherish the memories of our trip and the time we had together.

Once again, our deepest thanks and heartfelt appreciation for a very memorable visit to Philadelphia.

With deepest personal regards and best wishes for success and happiness.

Sincerely yours,
(Signature)
…, M.D.

12. 感谢邀请（Appreciation for being invited）

亲爱的 ×××博士：

作为 ××医学院院长，我代表我院全体教师和学生向您和您国家的人民伸出热诚的友谊之手。××医学院对您向我院副院长 ×××博士发出访问美国的邀请表示感谢。我感谢您为 ×××博士提供文化和学术交流的机会。

　　我们希望这次交流在某些方面能创造不同文化背景的人民之间的良好理解，并促进人民间的密切联系。

　　再次感谢您为实现我院人员访问美国提供的帮助。我们在承德将分享×××博士对这最激动人心的经历的期待，并羡慕他获此良机。

您的真诚的
×××博士

Feb. 2nd, 2017

..., Ph. D.
President
Univ. of New Jersey
Woodbury, N. J. 20098

Dear Dr. ...,

　　As President of ... Medical College, and on behalf of the faculty and students, I extend a warm hand of friendship to you and the people of your country. All of us appreciate the invitation extended by you to Dr. ..., Vice President of our college, to visit the United States. I wish to thank you for this opportunity offered to Dr. ... to share in this cultural and academic exchange.

　　We hope that this program, in some way, helps to create better understanding between people from different cultures and promotes a closer bond between our people.

　　Again, my appreciation for your assistance in making this opportunity available to one of our faculty. We, in Chengde, share in Dr, ... 's anticipation of this most exciting experience and envy the opportunity afforded him.

Sincerely yours,

(Signature)

…, M.D.

13. 感谢节日问候（Appreciation for greetings）

亲爱的×××博士：

感谢您寄来最近共进午饭时照的相片。我十分感谢×××博士为我们提供相识的机会。

××医学院为有您这样的贵客深感荣幸。我真诚希望这次相识是富有意义的，并使建立我们两校间的关系成为可能。

感谢您的周到考虑，向我们致以新年问候。我也希望您、您的家人及同事们新年快乐。

请告知我有关您来承德旅游的计划。如我什么时候去香港，一定去拜访您。

再次感谢您的友好而周到的接待。

您的真诚的

×××博士

Jan. 4, 2017

Dr. …

President

University of Hong Kong

Dear Dr. …,

Thank you so much for sending me the photos taken at our recent luncheon meeting. I am pleased that Dr. … provided us an opportunity to become acquainted.

… Medical College has been honored to have you as our guest. I do hope the experience has been a valuable one for you, and that it will be possible to enhance the relationship between our two universities.

I wish to thank you for your very thoughtful New Year's greeting and I want to wish you, your family and your colleagues, a very happy New Year.

Please keep me informed about your plans for further excursions to Chengde. If and when I travel to Hong Kong, I will surely see you again.

Thank you again for your continued friendship and thoughtfulness.

Sincerely,

(Signature)

…, M.D.

14. 感谢出席落成典礼（Appreciation for attending the dedication ceremony）

亲爱的×××教授：

感谢您最近的来信。知您平安返港，十分高兴。您来我院参加新建筑启用典礼，我们激动的心情无法形容。随信寄上一些相片，希望它能使您回忆起那愉快的时光。

再次感谢您赠给我们的珍贵礼品，它成为我院行政会议室新装饰的一部分，您带来的锦旗在那里显得格外漂亮。

欣闻贵校牙科医院将于2018年内落成，最使我们激动的是那时您将邀请我们参加落成典礼。我们盼望着那一天的到来，并为能再次见到您而感到欣慰。

请接受我对您和您的家人的良好祝愿。希望您们能再来承德访问。望保重身体，保持联系。

您的真诚的

×××博士

Jan. 28, 2017

Prof. ...
Dept. of Pathology
Green Mary Hospital
Univ. of Hong Kong

Dear Professor ...,

Thank you very much for your recent letter. I am delighted that you arrived safely back in Hong Kong. I can not tell you how much we enjoyed your participation in the dedication of our new building. Accompany this letter, please find some photographs which I hope will bring back pleasant memories to you.

Again I want to thank you for the lovely gift you brought. It is part of the new addition in the administrative conference room of our college. The banner you brought has something quite beautiful to view in its new addition.

I am delighted to hear that your new dental hospital will be dedicated sometime during 2018. Of course, I am extremely pleased that we are to receive official invitation to that event. We look forward to it very much and to the pleasure of seeing you again.

My very best wishes to you and your family. I hope that all of you will visit Chengde, again. Take good care of yourself and keep in touch with us.

Sincerely yours,
(Signature)
..., M.D.

第四节　申请信（**Application**）

　　有时为了取得学习机会、寻找工作以及参加会议等，根据有关信息，可写信去申请和应聘。申请信一般直接发到拟去学习或工作的单位。这类信件内容一般包括：

　　（1）介绍自己的简单情况，如：姓名、性别、年龄、某时某校毕业、专业情况、做过什么教学和科研工作。

　　（2）个人能力、学历、经历（也可附上本人履历表）。

　　（3）要求学习或工作的目的和时间，请求提供有关资料和入学（入会、求职）等表格。在最后一段可写上"希望早日得到您的答复"或"如能被接受，我将十分感谢"等词句。

1. 申请讲学（**Application to lecture**）

亲爱的 ××× 博士：

　　我是 ×× 医学院附属医院内科副教授。我写此信的目的是想向您表示，我愿在将来某个时候访问贵校。以前我曾到美国访问，受益匪浅。我很高兴地知道我们两校是姐妹学校，我愿意达成我们双方都可受益的某种计划。

　　能够到贵校讲学、参观、讨论和出席贵校的学术会议，都将令人激动。我所感兴趣的讲演题目是：病毒性肝炎的控制与诊断。

　　如果您对这个访问计划也感兴趣的话，请按以上地址同我联系。我将自己负担旅费，但希望您能提供住宿。即使我们不能达成这种协议，我将设法在我有机会赴美进行非官方访问时访问贵校。

　　非常感谢您为此事劳神和协助。

您的真诚的

××× 博士

..., M.D.

Dean

School of Medicine

East Carolina University

Greenville, North Carolina 27858

Dear Dr. ...,

　　I am an Associate Professor of Internal Medicine at ... Medical College Hospital. I am writing to express my interest in visiting your medical school sometime in the future. I traveled to the U. S. before and enjoyed my visit immensely. I was very pleased to learn that your medical school and my college have a "sister school" relationship. I would like to set up some kinds of programs that could be to our mutual benefit.

　　It would be very exciting to be able to come to your faculty and provide lectures, participate in discussions, and sit in on your conferences. My interests lie in the diagnosis and control of viral hepatitis.

　　If such a project is of interest to you also, please contact with me at the address above. I could pay my travel expenses, but would need housing. Even if we are unable to establish such contact. I will make an effort to visit your facility when I am in the U. S. for an unofficial visit.

　　Thank you very much for your time and assistance in this matter.

Sincerely yours,

(Signature)

..., M.D.

2.　申请教授针灸（Application to teach accupuncture）

亲爱的 ××× 博士：

　　我代表几所愿派毕业生到卡罗莱纳教一年或更长一段时间针灸的中国院校写这封信。我正计划从美国院校收集一些有关这方面需求的信息。

　　理想的是，愿去美国执教的人都经过专门训练，动机明确，无小孩拖累。他们唯一的希望是能为他们提供住宿和付给同普通美国医生的工资。

　　您能否提供一些有关贵院人员需求的信息？如能描述一下拟提供的住宿设施或介绍几位针灸专家的姓名，对我们也很有帮助。您提供的任何信息都将有助于促进学校和教师间相互联系。

　　盼望您的回复。

您的真诚的

××× 博士

Oct. 6, 2017

…, M.D.

President

East Carolina University

Greenville, North Carolina 27858

Dear Dr. …,

　　I represent several Chinese colleges that are interested in sending graduates to Carolina for a year or more to teach acupuncture. I am attempting to gather information from American colleges on their needs and requirements.

　　Ideally, the people interested in going to America would be

educated, motivated and without younger children. They would expect only housing and a wage paid to ordinary American doctors.

Could you give me some idea what your staffing need and requirements might be? It would also be helpful to have a description of available living facilities, or the names of acupuncture experts. Any information you can give to help put the school and the teachers in touch with one another would be helpful.

I look forward to hearing from you.

Sincerely,

(Signature)

…, M.D.

3. 申请转地进修（Application to transfer）

亲爱的 ××× 教授：

我1周前抵达费城，准备在宾夕法尼亚大学 ××× 教授的指导下做病毒性肝炎的控制和诊断的研究工作，但很不巧，××× 教授另有其他紧急任务，1年内不能指导我开展工作。

××× 教授建议我写信申请转到贵校，在您的指导下工作，因为您正做同类研究。同时，××× 教授还会向您写一封推荐信。宾夕法尼亚大学将协助办理我的转学手续。

如有幸从2017年10月至2018年7月在您的指导下做访问学者的工作，我将十分感谢。如能早得回信，不胜感激。

您的真诚的

×××

Sept. 3, 2017

Prof. ...

Yale University

New Haven, Connecticut

Dear. Professor ...,

    I arrived in Philadelphia a week ago to do research on the diagnosis and control of viral hepatitis with Professor ... of the University of Pennsylvania, but unfortunately, Professor ... will be involved in other urgent work for one year.

    Professor ... suggested that I should write to apply for a transfer to your university and work under your guidance since you are doing the similar work. Meanwhile, a letter of recommendation from Professor ... is being sent to you. The University of Pennsylvania will help with processing my transfer.

    I should be grateful to have the opportunity of working with you as a visiting scholar from October 2017 to July 2018. An early reply will be deeply appreciated.

Yours sincerely,

(Signature)

...

4. 申请进修（Application to study）

亲爱的先生：

    我写此信是想询问贵处是否接收外国访问学者。

    我今年46岁，是××医学院内科主治医师。我1995年毕业于××医学院，20年来在内科从事临床和教学工作。自2007年以来，我的研究题目是：急性心力衰竭、呼吸衰竭和肾衰竭，已发表了数篇论文。

我知道贵校抢救中心是世界闻名的。如您能考虑我到贵校这个专业进修和研究，我将感到非常荣幸。我的英文水平还不错，已通过了世界卫生组织举办的正式英语考试。现在，世界卫生组织将资助我到国外学习研究，就是说，它将为我提供生活费和往返机票。

我特别愿意到贵校的抢救中心工作，烦请您寄给我申请表和其他有关资料。如能接受我作为贵校访问学者，我将十分感谢。

随信附上我的履历表供您参考，盼望早日收到您的回信。

> 您的真诚的
>
> ×××博士

Aug. 8, 2017

University Health Care Center
University of Pittsburgh
Pittsburgh, PA 15260

Dear Sir,

I am writing to inquire if you accept visiting scholars from outside the U.S.

I am 46 years old, attending doctor of Internal Medicine at ... Medical College. I graduated from ... Medical College in 1995, and have been engaged in clinical and teaching work in Internal Medicine for more than 20 years. My research has been in diseases of acute heart failure, respiratory failure and renal failure since 2007, and the results have been published.

I know that your Critical Care Unit is well-known in the world, and I would be honored, were you consider me for further study and research in this field at your university. My English is reasonable and I have passed an official English examination given by WHO. Now I have a WHO sponsorship to do research and study abroad. That is, WHO will provide me with a stipend and round trip air tickets.

I am particularly interested in the ICU at your university and would like you to send me an application form and any other relevant information. I would be grateful if you could accept me as a visiting scholar in your University.

Enclosed is my Curriculum Vitae for your reference. I look forward to hearing from you soon.

Sincerely yours,
(Signature)
..., M.D.

5. 申请做科研工作（Application for research）

亲爱的 ×××博士：

许多年轻的中国学者愿意同美国学者一起做研究工作，他们来自文艺到科技的各个领域，每个人都是合格的专业人员。

我写此信是想得到一些信息以帮助我的同事寻找职位。烦请提供所附调查表列举的有关贵校的详细资料，以便让这些胜任各种工作的学者们能做好去美国生活和工作的准备。

这些人可适应各种文化环境，并渴望学习科学、技术、文化和其他有关医学教育和研究方面的先进技能。

我请求您帮助把他们介绍给贵校以及您们城市的有关单位。

您的真诚的
×××博士

Aug. 24, 2017

..., Ph. D.

Chairman

Dept. of Physiology

The Univ. of New York

New York, N. Y. 10024

Dear Dr. ...,

Many young Chinese scholars are interested in doing research with American Scholars. They are from different fields ranging from the art to science and technology. Each is highly qualified in their academic fields.

I am writing to you to obtain information that will help my colleagues in their search for positions. Therefore, some detailed information about your school is requested in the enclosed questionnaire so that qualified scholars can prepare for living and working in the U.S.

These people are very adaptable to different cultures and are eager to learn scientific, technical, cultural and other advanced skills in medical education and research work.

We are asking for your help to introduce them to your school and to the city in which it is located.

Sincerely yours,

(Signature)

..., M.D.

6. 申请攻读博士学位（Application for Ph. D.）

亲爱的×××博士：

我现在是××医学院五年制医学生，我将在 2017 年 8 月初毕业，并获医学学士学位。

我的志愿是从医，但我首先希望在美国一所大学获得哲学博士学位。

　　如果您愿意了解我更多的情况，如教育资格、语言技能或工作经历，或还需要我的其他个人情况，请通知我，我将把这些材料尽早寄上。

　　我也期待着您按本信地址寄给我有关资料。

　　感谢您费心关照。

您的真诚的

×××

…, M.D.

Dept. of Internal Medicine

The Univ. of Texas Hospital

Bellaire, Texas 77401

Dear Dr. …,

　　I am currently a five–year medical student at … Medical College, and will graduate in early August of 2017 with a B.S. degree.

　　I wish to pursue a career in medicine, but first I hope to obtain a Ph. D. degree from an institution in the United States.

　　If you would like any more information concerning my educational qualifications, language skill, or work experiences, or if you require personal references, please inform me, and these will be made available to you at the earliest possible time.

　　I respectfully request any information that you can forward for me at the above address.

　　Thank you for your time and consideration.

Sincerely yours,

(Signature)

…

7. 写信联系英国某地课程（Writing for a place on a course in England）

亲爱的先生：

请赐寄进入贵校研究生院的申请表以及其他您认为是我所必需的资料。我想 2016 年春开始攻读卫生学硕士学位。

2015 年 7 月，我将毕业于武汉医科大学，获学士学位，有望名列班级前茅。我还参加了我系指导老师黄博士所写的几篇论文的准备工作。此外，我确有信心能在今年 10 月和 12 月分别通过 TOEFL 和 GRE 考试。肯定我将来学习不会有太大的语言障碍。

您忠实的

林一山

Dear Sir,

I would like to ask you to send me the application forms for the Graduate School and any other pertinent information that you think necessary to me. I am interested in beginning to work toward a Master's Degree in Hygiene in the spring of 2016.

In July of 2015, I will graduate from Wuhan Medical University with a Bachelor's Degree in Hygiene at the top of my class. I have also participated in the preparation of several papers written by my faculty advisor, Dr. Huang. In addition, I an sure that I shall pass TOEFL and GRE in October and December this year respectively, while pursuing my studies I will have little trouble with a language barrier.

Sincerely yours

Lin Yishan

8. 申请奖学金（Application for scholarship）

亲爱的先生：

现在我是中国××医学院五年制医学生，我希望攻读生理学研究生学位。在明年夏天毕业之前，我将收集有关美国大学的资料。

我知道许多美国大学设有奖学金，但我不知道怎样申请。我衷心地希望您能为我提供贵校有关基金、住宿等方面的信息。

中国和美国正在又一次以前所未有的速度和活力来发展他们之间的传统友谊。我之所以希望得到您的帮助和信息，是希望能够得到只有美国才能给予的科学技术训练，把它带回国内以实现中国的卫生事业现代化。

对您给予的关注感激不尽。

您的真诚的

×××

Aug. 7, 2017

University Health Care Center
University of Pittsburgh
Pittsburgh, PA 15460

Dear Sir,

Presently I am a five-year student at ... Medical College, China, and wish to pursue postgraduate studies in physiology. Before graduating in the coming summer, I am beginning to gather information about American Universities.

I understand that many American Universities offer scholarships but I have no idea how to apply for one. I respectfully request your kindness in supplying me as much information as you have regarding available funds, housing, etc.

China and the United States are once again developing their traditional friendship at a rate and with a vigour never seen before. I am requesting your help and information in the hope that will be able to acquire skills in science and technology offered only in your country, which can be brought back to aid China in the modernization of health care.

My sincere appreciation for your consideration,

Yours sincerely,
(Signature)
…

9. 申请资助（Application for financial aid）

亲爱的 ×××博士：

未能及时回复您 2016 年 4 月 28 日的来信非常抱歉，因为我们同承德市文教委员会和坐落于北京的教育部商谈批准×××博士延长在神户大学学习的申请花了很长时间。不幸的是，由于缺少资金，教育部否决了×××的申请。××医学院也没有外汇能为 ×××博士提供在日本的生活费用。如果您或×××教授能在日本找到适当的科研奖学金来资助×××博士下一年度的最低生活费，她就能在神户大学再学习一年。

我衷心地希望这件事能合理解决。但不管怎样，我都应感谢您提供的任何帮助。

您的真诚的
×××博士

Jan 25, 2017

..., M.D.

Dept. of Neurosurgery

Neurological Institute

Kobe Univ.

Japan

Dear Dr. ...,

　　Forgive this belated reply to your kind letter of April 28, 2016, but it takes time to negotiate with the Cultural and Educational Committees of Chengde Municipality and Ministry of Education in Beijing for an official sanction of Dr. ... 's application for extending his term of study in Kobe University. Unfortunately the Ministry of Education has rejected Dr. ... 's application because of a lack of financial resources. ... Medical College has no foreign currency to provide living expenses for Dr. ... in Japan. If you or Professor ... could find an appropriate research fellowship grant in Japan which would provide minimal living expenses for another year, Dr. ... could remain in Kobe University.

　　I sincerely hope for an equitable solution, but in any case, you have my gratitude for any help you can give.

Sincerely yours,

(Signature)

..., M.D.

10. 申请参观访问（Application for visiting）

亲爱的 ××× 博士：

　　作为一名 ×× 医学院的行政官员，自 2008 年以来，我已经带领几批医务人员到美国学习医疗保健工作。我们访问过医院、诊所、公司和培养医务人员的教育研究机构。

在美国杂志上曾看到贵院在医学教育方面成就突出，我非常想带一个团组到贵院参观，学习有关医学教育体制的一些情况。这个团组里有护士、口腔医师、口腔保健医生、口腔技师和内科医生。

我希望我们多利用一些时间进行交流，整个访问时间大约半天以内。我们在萨克拉门托访问日期大约在6月15日至16日。

请回信，以便我们能继续安排我这个团组的活动日程。能事先安排好访问日程，我们双方都会感到满意。

感谢您的大力协助。

您的真诚的

×××

Jan. 26, 2017

..., Ph. D.

Assistant Dean

Allied Health Division

Sacramento City College

3825 Freeport Boulevard

Sacramento, CA 95822

Dear Dr. ...,

　　As an administrator from ... Medical College, I have, since 2008, brought groups of health personnel to America to study health care practices. We have visited hospitals, clinics, companies and educational institutes for medical personnel.

I have read in the American journals that your college has done good job in medical education, and would like very much to bring a group to tour your facility and learn something about the educational system. The group will consist of nurses, dentists, dental hygienists, dental assistants, and physicians.

It is my hope that we will have sufficient time to exchange ideas. The whole visit probably would not exceed a half day. The approximate date of our visit in Sacramento is June 15–16.

Please respond so that I may continue to plan for my group activities. With advanced planning, the visit can be enjoyable for both you and my group.

Thank you for your assistance.

Sincerely,

(Signature)

...

11. 申请职位（Application for position）

亲爱的 ×××博士：

　　我申请到贵校任职或做研究工作。我是 ×××医学院公共卫生系讲师。

　　随信附履历一份。如您能提供任何信息，我将不胜感激。

　　谨致问候。

您的真诚的

×××

May 24, 2016

Dr. ...
Chairman
Dept. of Biochemistry
Columbia University
New York, N. Y. 10049

Dear Dr. ...,

I am writing to apply for work or a research position at your University. I am a lecturer of the Public Health Department, ... Medical College.

Enclosed is a resume of my education and experience. Any information you can provide will be deeply appreciated.

With kind regards,

Sincerely yours,
(Signature)
...

12. 索要求职表（Asking for an application form for a post）

亲爱的先生：

我在 6 月 27 日《英国医学杂志》中看到一则有关贵院儿科招聘主治医师的广告。如能寄给我一份申请表将不胜感激。

您的忠实的
恩·康医生

5 Margery Terrace

Durham DH1 26Q

28 June, 2017

The Medical Staffing Officer

St George's Hospital

London SW1

Dear Sir,

I should be most grateful if you would send me an application form for the post of Registrar in the Department of Paediatrics as advertised in the *British Medical Journal* of 27th June.

Yours faithfully

N Khan (Dr)

13. 申请高级主治医师职务（Application for the post of senior registrar）

亲爱的先生：

我欲申请贵院在《英国医学杂志》（10月23日版）广告栏中登出的儿童精神病高级主治医师职务。

按要求呈上我的履历和3份证明书。

您的忠实的

欧玛·马硕德医生

62 Coverdale Crescent
London NW 3
26 October

The medical Staffing Officer
Whittington Hospital
Highgate Hill
London N19

Dear Sir,

　　I wish to apply for the post of Senior Registrar in Child Psychiatry as advertised in the *British Medical Journal* of 23th October.

　　I enclose my curriculum vitae and copies of three testimonials as requested.

Yours faithfully,
Omar Massoud (Dr)

14. 申请药剂师职务（Application for a position of pharmacist）

广州中山医科大学
药学系四年级 1 班
邮政编码：510089
2017 年 4 月 29 日

香港
玛丽娅医院
人力资源部

先生：

　　我是个中国人，祖籍为广东台山县。我父母在香港定居已经 30 年了,因而我已获得香港当局的许可去香港定居。我今年 7 月将从广州中山医科大学毕业。我主修的专业是药学,如果可能的话,我想于毕业之前在香港找定一份工作。

我早就希望毕业后为贵院工作,因为我认为贵院是香港最好的医院。我敢肯定,如果我有幸在贵院药房工作,我的知识和经验将会大大增加。

毋容置疑,在 7 月毕业之前,本人将修完药学方面一整套的普通课程。此外,我还选修了我们学校开设的在医院药剂方面的所有课程。我之所以这样做,是因为我一直就想当一名医院的药剂师。

随函附寄我的个人简历及 3 封推荐信。要是贵院在我毕业之时有空缺,如蒙考虑我的申请,本人将不胜感激。如届时无空缺,请将我的名字存档,因为我认为贵院的药房在香港是最好的。十分感谢您们的关照。

×××谨上

The Senior Class 1
Department of Pharmacy
Zhongshan Medical University
Guangzhou 510089
April 29, 2017

Human Resources Department
Maria Hospital
Hong Kong

Gentlemen:

I am a Chinese whose native place is Taishan County, Guangdong. My parents have been citizens of Hongkong for thirty years and I have got the approval from Hongkong authorities to settle down in

Hongkong. I will graduate from Zhongshan Medical University in Guangzhou this coming July. My major is Pharmacy and I wish to secure a position in Hongkong before I graduate, if possible.

I have long been in hope of working for you after graduation, because I consider you the finest hospital in Hongkong. I am sure that if I have the privilege of serving in your pharmacy, I will greatly increase my knowledge and my experience.

Needless to say, I will have completed a standard course in pharmacy before I graduate in July. In addition, I have chosen to elect all the courses available at my university in Hospital Pharmacy. I did this because I have all the time wanted to be a hospital pharmacist.

Attached with this letter are my curriculum vitae and three letters of recommendation. If you have a position available upon my graduation, I would appreciate your considering my application. If not, please keep my name on file, because I consider your pharmacy the best in Hongkong. Thank very much for your attention.

Yours sincerely,

(Signature)

…

15. 申请推迟开始上班的日期（Application to postpone the commencement of duties）

亲爱的先生：

感谢您 2017 年 3 月 3 日的来信，提供我由 2017 年 3 月 23 日起任贵院高级住院医生的工作。

非常高兴接受这一职务，但恰在 2017 年 3 月 1 日的面试后，我收到家中的电话，得知家父突然去世，母亲又患病。作为家中长子，我需返回巴基斯坦亲自料理后事。不知您能否为我推迟至 2017 年 4 月 1 日开始上班以允许我返回卡拉齐一趟？

如蒙予以考虑，将不胜感激。恭请赐复。

您的忠实的

纳希尔·加里尔医生

3 March, 2017

Professor Chocks

Department of Cardiology

St Thomas' Hospital

London SE1

Dear Sir,

Thank you for your letter of 3th March, 2017, offering me the post of Senior House Officer in Medicine from 23th March, 2017.

I am very pleased to accept the post but just after the interview on 1st March, 2017, I received a call from my family telling me that my father had died suddenly and my mother is ill. As the eldest son of the family it is necessary for me to return to Pakistan to make necessary arrangements. Would it, therefore, be possible for you to postpone the commencement of my post to 1st April, 2017, to allow me to travel to Karachi?

I should be most grateful if you would consider this and await your reply.

Yours faithfully

Nasir Jalil (Dr)

16. 申请入会（Application to join a society）

亲爱的先生：

自 2006 年以来，我一直是中华医学会生理学会会员。自医学院毕业25年来,我曾编著了有关生理及其他学科的2本书,发表了5篇论文。为了向更有造诣的同事们学习,求得指导、合作和协作,在生理学领域赶上迅速发展的形势,我申请加入贵会。

如您能惠寄入会须知和申请表,我将不胜感激。

非常感谢您对我的请求的关注。

您的真诚的

× × ×

Oct. 18, 2016

The Secretary

The Newton Physiology Society

Dear Sir,

Since 2006, I have been a member of the Physiology Society of Medical Association of China. In the 25 years since my graduation from medical school, I have written two books and five papers on physiology and other subjects. In order to learn from senior colleagues, to obtain their guidance, cooperation and coordination, and to keep up with the rapidly developing situation in physiology, I am applying for membership in your Society.

I shall be much obliged if you will be kind enough to provide me with a copy of your regulations together with an application form.

Your prompt attention to my request will be highly appreciated.

Sincerely yours,

(Signature)

...

17. 请求某人允许用其名字为推荐人（Asking for permission to use someone's name as a referee）

亲爱的怀特豪斯先生：

　　兹申请在贵院任高级主治医师职务,过去3个月中我曾在贵院工作过。如蒙允许用您的名字作为我的推荐人将万分感激。

您的忠诚的

曼里欧·贵德蒂医生

Department of Neurosurgery

Whittington Hospital

Highgate Hill

London N19

2 December, 2017

A B Whitehouse FRCS

Department of Neurosurgery

Royal Hospital

Glasgow

Dear Mr. Whitehouse,

I am applying for the post of Senior Registrar at the above hospital where I have been working for the past three months. I should be most grateful if you would allow me to use your name as a referee.

Yours sincerely

Manlio Guidetti (Dr)

第五节 推荐信（Recommendation）

推荐信是受某人之托来介绍某人情况的信函。推荐人同被推荐人的关系应该是熟悉的。推荐信的内容一般包括：与被推荐人的关系和相识时间，被推荐人的学历、经历、个人能力、学习情况、科研情况、长处、性格等。内容要真实、可靠。最后在信尾时要写上"希望推荐能被考虑"和"如能被接受，十分感谢"等词句。

1. 推荐做研究工作（Recommendation for research）

亲爱的 ××× 教授：

获悉您已接受 ××× 大夫到贵系做研究工作的申请，十分高兴。

我愿意向贵系推荐 ××× 大夫，他于 2008 年毕业于 ×× 医学院，并在我直接指导下完成了住院医师的训练。目前，他是内分泌组的主治医师。他在进行临床研究的同时，还在生化研究室进行代谢性骨病和各种内分泌疾病的镁代谢研究工作。

我发现他是位聪明、勤奋而富有求知欲的医生。在普通内科学和临床内分泌学方面，他知识相当丰富，但他需要更多的实验经验，以便他能胜任克汀病的临床研究工作。尽管我不能保证他英语讲得十分流利，但我相信，在短时期内他会克服这个困难。我知道，您既是药理学教授，也是医学教授。我一直渴望能有几位具有多种学科知识的助手。

我完全清楚，您明年的经费会有所裁减，我们的情况也是如此，但我仍然希望您能为 ××× 医生提供食宿，帮他实现远大的抱负。

致以衷心的问候。

您的真诚的

×××博士

May 21, 2017

Prof. ...

Dept. of Pharmacology

School of Medicine

The Johns Hopkins University

Baltimore, Maryland 21205

Dear Professor ...,

I am very glad to learn that Dr. ... 's application for a research fellowship in your department has received your favorable consideration.

It is my pleasure to recommend Dr. ... to your department. Dr. ... graduated from ... Medical College in 2008, and received full residency training in the department of medicine under my direct supervision. He is now an attending physician in the division of endocrinology. He has been working on the magnesium metabolism in metabolic bone disorders and various endocrine disease in the biochemical laboratory while carrying out clinical studies.

I find him to be an intelligent and industrious doctor with an inquiring mind. His knowledge of general medicine and clinical endocrinology is more than adequate, but he needs more laboratory experience to enable him to carry out the clinical investigation work of cretin. I can not guarantee him fluency in English but believe that he can overcome this difficulty in a short period. I understand that you are the professor of pharmacology as well as the professor of medicine. I have been longing to have a few assistants trained in multiple disciplines.

I fully understand that your budget for the coming year is being cut considerably. The same is true with us. But still I sincerely hope you can find a way to accommodate Dr. ... and help him to realize his ambition.

With kindest regards, I am.

Sincerely yours,
(Signature)
..., M.D.

2. 推荐出国进修（Recommendation for advanced study abroad）

亲爱的×××教授：

我写信向您推荐××医学院传染病研究室主治医师×××医生。他于2009年毕业于××医学院，尔后考取研究生，从事传染病研究，并于2012年获硕士学位。

×××医生是一位出色的学生，又是一位有培养前途的医生。我相信，如果您能接受他的话，他将是您系里最好的学生之一。他的英语不错，并通过了我国政府的官方考试，以取得政府资助出国学习和研究的资格。换言之，中国政府将为他提供奖学金和来往旅费。如您能接受他作为访问学者在您系工作，我将感激不尽。

盼望您早日答复。

您的真诚的
×××博士

August 30, 2017

Prof. …

Dept. of Clinical Microbilolgy

Karolinska Sjukhuset

Box 60500, 10401 Stockholm

Dear Professor …,

I am writing to introduce to you Dr. …, who is a visiting doctor at the Institute of Infectious Diseases, … medical College.

He graduated from … Medical College in 2009 and continued his postgraduate work in infectious diseases, receiving the Master's Degree in 2012.

Dr. … was an excellent student, and has boundless prospects as a doctor. I am confident that he could be one of the best students in your department if he were accepted. His English is good, and he has passed an official English examination given by our government. He now qualifies for government sponsorship to do research and studies abroad. That is, the Chinese government will provide him with a stipend and round trip airfare. I would be grateful if you could accept him as a visiting scholar in your department.

I look forward to hearing from you at the earliest possible moment.

Sincerely yours,

(Signature)

…, M.D.

*　　　*　　　*

亲爱的 ××× 教授：

我非常高兴地写信向您推荐 ××× 先生。在 ×× 医学院,我们都以×××的研究成果和教学经验而自豪。在我系的发展中,以及在使我系重新成为科学先进、学术优秀的集体的过程中,我们也为他的聪明才智感到骄傲。

自2003年到医学院工作之日起,×××就在教学和实验研究工作方面孜孜不倦的工作,以努力获得建设新中国所必须的现代技术,并把它传授给同事们和学生们。

由于×先生十分谦虚,我想他不会告诉您,他在甲状腺肿理论方面的几篇论文已获国家奖,而且有些技术和理论已被全国各医院、研究所和大专院校采用。

除此之外,与×××先生共事令人愉快。他工作勤奋,助人为乐,心地善良,体贴同事和学生。我可断定,我们系没有一个人比他做的贡献更多。我们盼望他有机会出国深造,回国后帮助我们增进知识,完善机构,改进科研和教学方法。

我们为他离去两年而遗憾,但我们想,您可以从他那里大有所得,而我们又将从您那里受益更多。

我们衷心希望您会给我们一个满意的答复。

您的真诚的

×××博士

April 30, 2017

Prof. …
University Hospital
Dept. of Biomedical Engineering
The University of Washington

Dear Professor …,

I am delighted to have been asked to write a letter of recommendation for … . We, here at … Medical College, are very proud of his research, his teaching, and his intelligent help in developing and reshaping our department into a unit aimed at achieving scientific and academic excellence.

Since his arrival here in 2003, ... has worked ceaselessly through both his teaching and laboratory research to acquire and pass on to colleagues and students the modern technology essential to building New China.

Mr. ..., I am sure, is too modest to tell you that several of his papers on goiter theory have won national acclaim here in China, and some of his techniques and theories have been adopted for use throughout Chinese hospitals, research institutes and universities.

Besides all this, it is a pleasure to work with Mr. ... .. He is always hardworking, helpful, kind and considerate of colleagues and students. I can firmly say that no one in our department has made greater contributions than he, and it is our ardent desire that he have an opportunity to study abroad so that he can improve our knowledge, our organization and our research and teaching methods on his return.

We are sorry to lose him even for two years, but we think you will gain a great deal from his presence at your University and that we, in turn, will gain from you.

We sincerely hope your decision in his case is a favorable one.

Yours truly,
(Signature)
..., M.D.

3. 推荐攻读学位（Recommendation for a degree）

亲爱的 ××× 博士：

我非常高兴地向您推荐我以前的学生 ××× 先生。他正向贵校寻求攻读博士学位的机会。

×××先生于2008年至2012年在××医学院生物医学工程系电子仪器和自动测量技术专业学习。他聪明、勤奋并乐于助人。

他学习过高级英语,并在英语竞赛中获奖。他总是班上三位最好的学生之一,并于2011至2012年获得了奖学金。×××先生的实验也做得相当出色。他的毕业论文成绩为"A",当时仅有几个学生达到"A"级水平。

我希望上述情况使您能对×先生的能力有一个较好的印象,我也愿意回答您今后提出的任何问题。

如蒙接收,感激不尽。

您的真诚的

×××博士

April 4, 2017

..., M.D.

Dean

School of Medicine

Univ. of California

Los Angles, CA 20098

Dear Dr. ...,

I am very pleased to recommend my former student, Mr. ..., who is seeking admission to the Ph. D. program at your institute.

Mr. ... studied at the Electronic Instruments and Automatic Measurement Technique Division of the Biomedical Engineering Department at ... Medical College during 2008–2012. Mr. ... is intelligent, hardworking and always enjoys helping others.

He studied advanced English and won prizes in English competition. He was always among the top three students in all of his classes. He received a scholarship of … Medical College in 2011 and 2012. Also, Mr. … distinguished himself in his experimental work. He received an "A" on his graduate thesis, being one of a few students who did so.

I hope the above information will give you a fair picture of Mr. … 's ability, but I will be glad to answer any further inquiry you might have.

Your acceptance of Mr. … will be deeply appreciated.

Sincerely yours,
(Signature)
…, M.D.

4. 推荐转学（Recommendation for transferring to other college）

亲爱的 ××× 教授：

我非常高兴地向您推荐 ××× 博士。她是 ×× 医学院病生理学讲师，也是我院附属医院急救中心负责人。自 2000 年毕业于医学院以后，她一直在病理生理教研室从事教学与科研工作。近年来，她还从事临床危重患者的弥漫性血管内凝血的研究工作。

今年 11 月，她将完成在加拿大安大略大学麻醉系的学习。她希望到您的急救中心继续学习。如您能接收她为访问学者到贵中心学习 3 至 6 个月，我将不胜荣幸。

我认为 ××× 博士是一位前途远大而诚实的同事，并相信她完全能胜任您的工作。

致以良好的问候。

您的真诚的
××× 博士

Sept. 18, 2017

Prof. ...

President of International Centre

The Cleveland Clinic Foundation

9500 Euclid Avenue

Cleveland, Ohio 44106

Dear Professor ...,

I take great pleasure in introducing you Dr. ..., lecturer of pathophysiology at ... Medical College and Director of the Intensive Care Unit of College Hospital. She graduated from ... Medical College in 2000, and has been doing teaching and research work in the department of pathophysiology. She has also been working, in recent years, in the hospital wards on the problem of disseminated intravascular coagulation of critically ill patients.

By November this year, she will finish her study in Department of Anesthesia, Ontario University Hospital, London, Ontario, Canada. She intends to go to your ICU to pursue further study. I would consider it a great favour if you could accept her as a visiting scholar for a period of three to six months in your Intensive Care Unit.

I have found Dr. ... to be a promising and sincere colleague. I am sure that she is fully qualified to serve as one of your assistants during her visit there.

With best regards,

Sincerely yours,

(Signature)

..., M.D.

5. 推荐出国讲学（Recommendation for presenting lecture abroad）

亲爱的 ××× 博士：

我十分荣幸地代表 ×× 医学院为两位能干而受人尊敬的同事写信给您。

今年6月，××× 医生将要结束4年的内科住院医师的工作。在内科工作时，他无论在照料病人方面，还是在辅导其他医生和学生方面，都显出卓越的才华。××× 医生是 ×× 医学院的本科生，在 ×× 医学院获得硕士学位。多年的学习使他知识渊博。

××× 夫人在 ×× 医学院附属医院从事了4年的护理工作。她取得了护理学学士学位。作为高级护师，她对教育其他护士，参加为新毕业生和护理系学生而安排的护理教育规划活动表现出极大的兴趣，最近已被提升为心肺复苏科的负责人。××× 夫人工作效率高，感情细腻，是一位职业护理工作者。

××× 医生和他夫人将成为贵校的宝贵财富，他们乐于与您们交流知识并向您们学习。我极力向您推荐他们，并希望他们能在加拿大工作，这对各方面来说都是有益的。

您的真诚的

×××

March 27, 2017

… M.D.

Dean and Vice President

School of Medicine

University of Western Ontario

London, Canada N6A, 5A5

Dear Dr. …,

It is an honour for me to write on behalf of two very capable and highly respected individuals affiliated with … Medical College.

This June, Dr. … will complete a four-year residency in internal medicine. Throughout his training in internal medicine, he has displayed excellence in both patient care and the ability to teach other physicians and medical students. Dr. … attended … Medical College as an undergraduate and attained his Master's degree from … Medical College. He has been a high achiever throughout his years of study.

Mrs. … has been a nurse at … Medical College Hospital for four years. She is a graduate of our College's Baccalaureate Nursing Program. As a staff nurse, she has shown great interest in educating her fellow nurses by participating in our nursing program for new graduates and nursing students, and lastly by becoming an instructor of cardiopulmonary resuscitation. Mrs. … is a professional and delivers nursing care with proficiency and sensitivity.

Dr. and Mrs. … could prove to be a great asset to your Medical College. They are eager to share their knowledge and to learn from your staff. I highly recommend them to you and hope that their stay in Canada will be a rewarding experience for everyone.

Sincerely,
(Signature)
…, M.D.

6. 推荐出国访问（Recommendation for a visit）

亲爱的×××博士：

您已获悉我院口腔医院×××博士将于2016年12月下旬至2017年1月上旬去美国访问。

为了保持我们的学术联系，我向您推荐×××博士到德克萨斯大学口腔医院为教师和学生们讲学，内容涉及普通牙科学的各个方面，包括传染性危害和局部义齿。

　　×××博士的普通牙科学知识非常丰富，而且表现出色。我相信，他将为您的工作计划做出令人满意的贡献，并希望他有可能参加您的讲学活动。

　　我为两校的友好关系而感到高兴，并盼望着有一个对贵方和我方都颇有益处的未来。

您的真诚的
×××博士

July 10, 2016

..., M.D.
Department of General Practice
University of Texas
Texas Medical center
Houston, Texas 77225

Dear Dr. ...,

You are aware that Dr. ... of the Dental Hospital of our College will visit the United States during the latter part of December and early part of January, 2016–2017.

It is my recommendation, in keeping with our academic affiliation, that Dr. ... present lectures to the students and faculty of the Dental School of the University of Texas on various aspects of general dentistry, including infectious hazards and removable partial dentures.

Dr. ... is well versed in the subject of general dentistry, and presents himself quite well. I am confident that he will make a significant contribution to your program and hope that it will be possible for him to participate in your lecture program.

I am pleased with the relationship between our two institutions, and look forward to a mutually beneficial future for both of us.

Sincerely,
(Signature)
..., M.D.

7. 推荐参加学术会议（Recommendation to attend a congress）

亲爱的 ×××博士：

我十分高兴地代表我 ××医学院的同事 ×××博士写信给您，他想参加 2017 年 9 月在洛杉矶举行的第二届美洲心脏病学会会议。

×××博士是研究心脏钙代谢的专家。他希望在这次会议上宣读一篇论文。如果您能给他发一封邀请信，我将十分感谢。他的通信地址是：

中华人民共和国　河北省承德市
××医学院　心脏科
×××,医学博士

十分感谢您对他表示的友好情意。您可以直接写信与他商讨出席会议的可能性。

致以个人的友好问候。

您的真诚的
×××博士

Jan. 10, 2017

..., Ph. D.
President
The University of Washington
Washington, D. C. 20016

Dear Dr. ...,

It is a pleasure to write on behalf of my colleague, Dr. ... from ... Medical University, who intends to attend the 2nd ACA Congress to be held in Los Angeles in September, 2017.

Dr. ... is an expert in the area of calcium metabolism in the heart and would be very happy to give a paper on the subject at the Congress. I would greatly appreciate it if it were possible for you to extend an invitation for him. His address is:

..., M.D.
Dept. of Cardiology
... Medical University
Chengde, Hebei Province
The People's Republic of China

Many thanks for any courtesy that you can extend to Dr. ... . You may write directly to him regarding the possibility of his presentation.

With worm personal regards.

Sincerely yours,
(Signature)
..., M.D.

第六节 欢迎来访信(Welcome to Visit)

在欢迎某人或代表团来某地访问的信件中,要写出以下几点:

(1)欢迎某人或代表团到某地来访问、讲学、参加会议等,并说一些表示友好的词句。

(2)对到达时间、接站、住宿、会见、讲学、游览活动等安排加以说明。

(3)提出访问期间的费用问题。

(4)最后可写上一些热情盼望来访的词句。

1. 欢迎代表团来访(Welcome a delegation to visit)

亲爱的×××博士:

非常高兴收到您2017年7月14日的来信,得知您将要和您的一些同事们于11月来中国访问。从您的来信中,获悉您将访问高等院校以及医学院校。您已知道,我们是医学院校,可以为您提供有关中国医学教育各方面的材料。

如果您的代表团能利用约半天的时间与我院各方面人士就对您们团组至为重要的事项进行交谈,那就太好了。

我曾设法为您寻求资助,以支付您在承德的费用,但未获成功。我们经常邀请和招待来自许多国家的贵宾,无力承担所有代表团的费用,难以提供您所寻求的资助。

如果您在访问中认为仍有可能来承德访问,我将为您安排与教师们共同讨论您们感兴趣的问题。在这方面,如果您能将代表团特别感兴趣的问题提前告诉我,那将格外有益。

我期待着收到有关您访问计划的更多信息,希望能互相见面。

您的真诚的

×××博士

Aug. 10, 2017

..., Ph. D.
President
The University of Washington
Washington, D. C. 20036

Dear Dr. ...,

I was pleased to receive your letter of July 14, 2017 advising me that you and a group of your colleagues are planning to visit China in November. From the tone of your letter, it sounds as if your primary mission is to visit a variety of colleges and medical schools during the course of your visit in China. You are, of course, aware that we are a medical college, but we can provide you with information about various aspects of medical education in China.

We would be very pleased to have you spend half of the day or so talking with various members of our staff to address the issues and concerns of greatest importance to your group.

Unfortunately, my efforts to identify potential financial support for your expenses while in the city were not productive. While we frequently have the opportunity to invite and host various dignitaries from many countries, we do not have a budget to defray the expense of all the delegations; and hence cannot offer you the support you are seeking.

However, if you still find it possible to visit Chengde during your travels throughout China, I will be very pleased to arrange for a visit here to discuss your many interests with the members of our staff. In this regard, it would be particularly helpful if I might have some advance information about the specific question or issues in which your delegation would be most interested.

I look forward to receiving further information about your planned visit and hope that our paths cross.

Sincerely yours.
(Signature)
…, M.D.

2. 欢迎学生来学习（Welcome a student to study）

亲爱的 ×××先生：

非常高兴收到您的来信。您希望从 2017 年 10 月 1 日至 12 月 30 日来我们医院学习，我们表示欢迎。您可做一些临床工作和考察工作。您来学院后，将与我们附属医院的大夫们共同工作。医院里的每一科室都有一两名英语讲得好的大夫。从留学生宿舍到医院骑自行车需要 10 分钟。安顿好后您应去买辆自行车，因为高峰期间乘汽车到医院非常拥挤。学费每月 200 美元，根据您的选择，住宿费用每月 100 美元至 200 美元不等。自己付饭费，每天 2~3 美元。如果您计划在中国旅行，短途可乘火车，长途可乘飞机。一个城市的旅费大约为 150 美元，包括飞机或火车票以及食、宿。随信寄去 ×× 医学院的简介供您参考。

你决定来中国后，请通知我。然后我们给您寄去 ×× 市政府的邀请信，您可以在明年初到中国驻德国大使馆办理签证手续。

盼速回信。

您的真诚的
×××

Oct. 10, 2017

...

Durerstra Be 43

1000 Berlin 45

Dear Mr. ...,

I am pleased to have your letter asking for a medical clerkship in our hospital from October 1 to December 30, 2017.

You are welcome to participate in some clinical work as well as observe. Upon your arrival, you will work with doctors in our affiliated hospitals. In each department, there is one or two doctors who speak English quite well. It takes 10 minutes to travel by bicycle from the Dormitory for Foreign Students to our hospital, and you should plan to buy a bicycle after you settle down here, because it is very difficult to travel by bus to and from the hospital in the rush hours. Tuition is $200 per month. Lodging costs are $100 to 200 per month depending upon the room you will stay in. You must provide your own meals, which cost two or three dollars per day. If you intend to travel within China, you can take trains for short distances and airplane for far travel. The cost of traveling within China is about $150 for one city, including air of or train tickets, hotel and meals. I am enclosing a copy of introduction of ... Medical College for your reference.

Please let me know if you decide to come. We will send you a letter of invitation from the ... Municipal Government with which you can get your visa from the Chinese Embassy in Germany early next year.

I am looking forward to hearing form you soon.

Sincerely yours.

(Signature)

..., M.D.

3. 欢迎来校访问（Welcome to visit college）

亲爱的×××博士：

得知您今年8月将来中国，十分高兴。重要的是您需要告诉我到达北京的时间，我们好去机场接您。请告诉我您认为在哪里住比较方便，以下建议供您选择：

（1）您可以住在我院的外宾招待所；

（2）您可以住在宾馆；

（3）您可以住在留学生宿舍。

无论您住在哪里，我们都将为您免费提供。您将是我们以及我们学院的客人。这次一定要多停留几天，我们可以到北京或其他您愿意去的地方观光。我心情非常激动，急切地等待着有关您到达日期和时间的消息。

我已将您来访的消息转告给×××院长，他盼望着您的到来并计划为您准备一次丰盛的晚餐。

请不要带礼物来。的确没有必要。我们拥有最珍贵的礼物——友谊，以及它给予的感人肺腑的美好回忆。

对您的家人致以最热情的问候，盼望收到您的旅行计划。

您的真诚的

×××博士

July 17, 2017

Dr. ...

Director

Division of International Surgical

Education and Practice

Jefferson Medical College

Thomas Jefferson University

Philadelphia, 19107

Dear Dr. ...,

We are so happy that you will be coming to China in August. It is important that you let me know when you will arrive in Beijing for we will meet you at the airport. Also let me know where it is convenient for you to live. You have several options.

(1) You may live in the Building for Foreign Guests on our College campus

(2) Accommodations at hotel.

(3) You may live in the foreign student dormitory.

Whatever accommodations you choose, there will be no charge to you. You will be our guest and the College's. Please do stay long enough to spend some time with us, and perhaps take a trip to Beijing or a place of your choice. I am very excited and await news of your arrival date and time.

I told Dr. ..., President of our College that you are coming and he too looks forward to seeing you. He plans to take you for a fine dinner.

Please do not bring gifts—no necessary. We have the most wonderful gift—that of friendship and the heartful warm memories it provides.

With my warmest regards to your family, and anticipating the receipt of your travel plans.

Sincerely yours.
(Signature)
..., M.D.

* * *

亲爱的×××博士：

　　我已收到了您10月8日的来信以及您来访的初步计划,您的来访使我们非常高兴。

　　因为我是承德人,所以感到您计划在这里停留的时间太短了。您的代表团可能会对到几个大专院校去参观感兴趣。××大学是个非常杰出的大学,它包括理科、经济以及一个教师学院;××大学以其科学和技术闻名于中国。如果您希望参观任何一所或全部院校,我将为您做出适当的安排。我注意到您没安排去清东陵,并相信您知道承德到清东陵的路程是230公里,即使是一个短暂的参观也需要一天的时间。

　　××大学和××大学是中国的重点院校,您如有时间,可去参观一下。如您有兴趣,我可与那里的教授进行联系。

　　我11月29日星期四在北京。但是在您访问的其他时间里,我将在学校。我随时都高兴迎候您的代表团光临。

您的真诚的
×××博士

Oct. 19, 2017

..., M.D.

Professor and Chairman

Rockefeller University

New York, N. Y. 104468

Dear Dr. ...,

I have received your letter of October 8 along with your preliminary program. We are pleased to have you visit us.

Because I am born in Chengde, I feel that the time you are planning to spend in our city is too short. Your delegation might be interested in visiting several institutions here: ... University is an outstanding university with programs in many fields including science, economics and a teacher's college; ... University is a university famous for science and technology in our country. If you wish to visit any or all of these institutions, I will try to make appropriate arrangements for you. I note that East Ching Dynasty Tombs are not on your schedule. I am certain that you know that the East Ching Dynasty Tombs are about 230 km from Chengde, and even a short visit would require a full day.

... University and ... University are leading Chinese universities and perhaps you could find time to visit them. I could contact with the professors there if you are interested.

I will be in Beijing on Thursday, November 29 but will be in my college all the other days of your visit and would be pleased to meet with your delegation at your convenience for any period of time you wish.

Sincerely yours.
(Signature)
..., M.D.

4. 欢迎来校攻读学位（Welcome to study for degree）

亲爱的×××先生：

我们已经收到了您所有的申请表格，并从其他渠道得到全部必要的文件和材料。

所有材料的初审结果表明，您符合我院的录取资格。您将于2018年秋季参加研究生的课程学习，攻读医学学位。

我们真诚地欢迎您来我院学习。

您的真诚的
×××博士

Sept. 2, 2017

Dental Department
University of Penn.
Philadelphia, PA 19104

Dear Mr. ...,

　　We have received your completed application form and all the necessary documents and materials from other sources.

　　A preliminary check of the materials indicates that you are academically eligible for admission. We wish to inform you that you will be admitted into the graduate course of ... Medical College for the fall term 2018 to work towards the degree of medicine.

　　We heartily welcome you to join us on our campus.

Yours truly,
(Signature)
..., M.D.

第七节　商谈学术交流信
（Discussion of an Academic Exchange）

　　在双方商谈学术交流时,应该注意写明以下内容:
　　（1）提出学术交流的起因。
　　（2）进行学术交流的益处。
　　（3）进行学术交流的方法和规模。
　　（4）学术交流的组织和费用。
　　（5）学术交流的发展和未来。

1. 讨论交流项目（Discussion of an exchange program）

亲爱的×××博士：

　　×××博士已和我就您的来信进行了商谈，我完全赞同您提出的××医学院和西安大略大学进行交流的计划。

　　我们对来自贵校的交流人员表示欢迎，并将为他们承担在我院的生活费。我将鼓励我校人员接受您的邀请，去访问西安大略大学。

　　您邀请我作为两校的外交联络人员去访问贵校，对此我特别感激。

　　致以良好的问候和祝愿。

您的真诚的

×××

January 29, 2017

…, M.D.

Professor & Chairman

Department of Anaesthesia

The Univ. of Western Ontario

London, Canada N6A 5A5

Dear Dr. …,

　　Dr. … has discussed your correspondence with me and I am completely supportive of your plans to encourage an exchange of faculty between … Medical College and the University of Western Ontario.

　　Certainly we will be very pleased to welcome exchange visitors from your University to our College and provide assistance to cover their living expense while here. I will also encourage members of our

College to accept your invitation to visit the University of Western Ontario.

I am particularly grateful for your kind invitation to me to visit your university as diplomatic liaison between our two institutions.

With best regards and kind wishes,

Sincerely yours,

(Signature)

…

2. 讨论学者交流计划(Discussion of faculty exchange program)

亲爱的 ××× 博士:

收到您 2017 年 6 月 6 日的来信,得知 ××× 博士已平安返回休斯敦,甚为高兴。我完全支持您愿意与我院建立姐妹学校和鼓励两校人员交流的计划。您这一想法令人振奋。我认为,交流对我们两校都大有益处。

对我们来讲,应让有经验的以及年轻有为的人员作为访问学者去贵校学习。我十分赞同您的意见,即派出人员数量开始时要少。我们的建议是,两校各派出两名高级人员和两名青年骨干人员,时间为 2 至 4 周。在这期间,我们的科技人员学习和研究口腔临床工作,交流经验,并与贵校的同事们进行个人间的信息交流。

我们特别希望从口腔系或口腔医院派一、二名年轻有为的人员去学习或接受一、二年的训练。希望贵校能为他们提供往返旅费,并为他们在休斯敦安排住宿。我们当然欢迎贵校交流人员来承德和中国其他城市访问,访问与旅游所需的费用将由我校支付,并将由一位翻译陪同。我们衷心希望这些想法能得到您的支持,并取得圆满成功。

盼望收到您的回信。

您的真诚的

×××博士

June 20, 2017

Dr. ...

Dean

Dental Branch

The University of Texas

Houston, Texas 77225

Dear Dr. ...,

I was very pleased to receive your letter of June 6, 2017, informing me of Dr. ... 's safe return to Houston. I am completely supportive of the plans to establish a sister relationship with your school, and encourage an exchange of faculty between our two institutions. The idea is an exciting one. In my view, the exchange would provide great benefit to both of our institutions.

From our side it would be best initially to have our senior faculty and promising young scientists as exchange scholars. I quite agree with you that we should start off small in this regard. We suggest that two senior members and two young scientists from each of our institutions cross visit for a time span of perhaps 2 or 4 weeks. During this period our scientists would study and observe the practice of dentistry, exchange dental experiences, and enjoy a personal exchange of information with your colleagues.

We especially want to send one or two promising young dentists of our stomatology department and dental hospital to study or to be trained for a period of one or two years. We hope that you can provide round trip air tickets and arrange accommodations for their stay in Houston. We certainly would be very pleased to welcome exchange visitors from your institution to visit Chengde and other cities in China. All expenses for your visits and sightseeing, with the help of an interpreter, would be covered by our college. We sincerely hope that these ideas receive your support and can reach fruition.

I am looking forward to hearing from you.

Sincerely yours,
(Signature)
…, M.D.

3. 探讨交流项目的可能性（Exploring possibility of an exchange program）

亲爱的 ××× 博士：

您可能还记得，去年我和 ××× 先生有幸访问过贵校。

从通信地址中您可能已经注意到，我现在在距北京 240 公里的 ×× 医学院工作，×× 医学院在内分泌和神经病学领域的工作成绩出色。这些系的领导对与美国医学院校的交流表现出极大的兴趣。

我今年 10 月份将回到佛罗里达。得悉贵校名望很高，我愿借此机会与您及您的同事们共同探讨学者交流的可能性。

我 10 月 12 日、13 日和 14 日在坦帕做短暂停留，其间您如方便，我希望有机会与您会晤。

由于时间较紧，我们一到达即与您联系，商谈具体安排。

盼望再次见到您。

您的真诚的
××× 博士

Sept. 8, 2017

..., M.D.

Dean

School of Medicine

University of Florida

Tampa, Florida 33647

Dear Dr. ...,

You may recall that last year Mr. ... and I had the opportunity to visit your University.

As you can see from my address, I am now working in ... Medical College, 240 km from Beijing ... Medical College has an excellent record in the areas of endocrinology and neurology. The heads of these departments have expressed to me an interest in entering into a faculty exchange with an American medical institution.

Since I am returning to Florida in October of this year, and knowing of your institution's fine reputation, I would like to discuss with you and your associate the possibilities of such an exchange.

We will be in Tampa on October 12, 13 and 14. If it is convenient for you to meet us during our short visit to Tampa we would welcome the opportunity.

Since time is so short, we will get in touch with you upon our arrival regarding further arrangements.

We look forward to meeting with you once more.

Very truly yours,

(Signature)

..., M.D.

4. 探讨系际交流的可能性（Exploring possibility of a Dept. to Dept. exchange program.）

亲爱的×××教授：

　　两天前刚回国的×××教授已将您2016年12月20日的信转交给我，十分高兴得知您将到承德访问。

　　×××教授同我商谈了两校进行某种形式交流的可能性，特别是在生理学和生化方面的交流。我建议，作为开端，贵校生理学和生化学的教授可直接与我院生理教研室主任×××教授和生化教研室主任×××教授联系，告之您的提议的某些细节。

　　我愿在承德随时恭候您并进一步商谈。

　　致以最诚挚的个人问候。

您的真诚的

×××

Jan. 8, 2017

…, M.D.
President
University of Hong Kong
Hong Kong

Dear Prof. …,

　　Professor …, who arrived two days ago, has forwarded to me your kind letter of December 20, 2016. It will be a great pleasure to have you visit us on your next trip to Chengde.

　　Prof. … has discussed with me the possibility of establishing some form of exchange between our two institutions, especially in the fields of physiology and biochemistry. May I suggest that, as a beginning, your professors of physiology and biochemistry write directly to Prof. ..., Chairman of our Physiology Department and Prof. ..., Chairman of the Biochemistry Department giving them some details of your proposal?

I would be willing to meet with you any time in Chengde for further discussion.

With best personal regards,

Sincerely yours,
(Signature)
..., M.D.

5. 探讨校际交流的可能性(Exploring possibility of a school to school exchange program)

亲爱的 ××× 教授:

感谢您 7 月 12 日的来信,得知您非常希望来我院访问。这使我想到了您 6 月 17 日的来信,信中谈到了加利福尼亚大学和 ×× 医学院建立合作一事。这一想法令人振奋,对两校都将有益。问题是如何找到最好的方法进行交流。前几天,我和 ××× 博士就两校交流问题进行了一次长谈,他是贵校的内科专家,现在我校任教。我希望他能把我们的想法以及他个人对交流的想法转告给您。

我认为,对两校最有益的交流是实现更多的学者交流。就我们而言,最好是交换具有多年工作经验的师资。我有如下建议请您考虑是否可行。

我院的高级师资到加利福尼亚大学访问 2~4 周。其间,他们可以考察医学临床工作、讲学或举办讲座,并与贵校的同事们交流信息。

收到贵校院长或对交流感兴趣的系主任们的邀请信,有助于获得签证。我们希望贵校能为他们在洛杉矶安排食宿。除洛杉矶之外,他们还愿意参观旧金山和其他城市。我相信,贵校的同事们会帮助他们做出安排。

学术交流将加强我们两校的友谊,使我们对贵校有一个充分的了解,并导致合作项目的建立。

我希望这些想法能使我们的商谈更具体。我院×××副院长对这项交流很感兴趣。我知道,这需要我院各学术部门有力的支持。我们盼望听到您的建议和评论。

致以良好的问候。

您的真诚的

× × ×

July 26, 2017

…, M.D.

Professor & Chairman

Dept. of Medicine

University of California

Los Angeles, California 90024

Dear Prof. …,

Thank you for your letter of 12 July in which you so graciously indicated your desire to visit us here. This brings me to your letter of June 17th and your remarks about collaboration between the medical staff at the University of California and that of … Medical College. The idea is an exciting one and could be of mutual benefit. The difficulty is to find the best approach. A few days ago I had a long discussion on this very subject with Dr. …, a physician from your University who is teaching here now. I hope that he will convey to you our ideas as well as his own thoughts on this matter.

In my view, the exchange that would be most beneficial to both of our institutions would be one that makes more places available for exchange scholars. From our view, it would also be best to exchange senior faculty members. Please give me your views on the following ideas.

Senior members of our College would visit the University of California for a time span of perhaps 2 to 4 weeks, during which time, they would observe your practice of medicine, give lectures and seminars, and exchange information with their American colleagues.

An invitation from your Dean or Chairmen of interested departments would help to get visas. We would hope that you could arrange for their living accommodations in Los Angeles. In addition to Los Angeles, faculty from our College would likely visit San Francisco and other cities in the States, which, I am sure, can be arranged with the help of our American colleagues.

Such an arrangements for academic exchange would provide a closer relationship and a better understanding of our respective institutions and could lead to constructive collaborative projects.

I hope that these ideas move our discussions towards something more concrete. My Vice President, ..., M.D. is very interested in such a project, and I know that it would have the necessary support of our academic departments. We are looking forward to your suggestions and comments.

With best regards,

Sincerely yours,

(Signature)

.... M.D.

第八节   开业大夫给会诊医生的信
（Letter to Consultant from GP）

以下是一些开业医生（GPs）介绍病人去上级医院时的写信范例。撰写这类信函时，重要的是要写明病人的全名、出生日期和表现症状。对于非英文姓名，最好在姓氏下面划线，如果病人曾经去过该医院就诊，应加以说明，并尽可能提供其住院号或门诊号。

1. 左腹不适（Discomfort in the left abdomen）

亲爱的医生：

有关 Charles Oxley 26, 3, 42 (m) 42 Liverpool Way N14

该病人主诉间断腰背痛已 2 年之久，近来又隐约感到左腹不适。此症状与进食与否无关。大小便正常。骨科检查发现病人脊柱活动受限。腹部无异常发现。腹痛大概起因于脊柱病变，谨此特请您高诊，不胜感激。

您的忠实的

Michael Apostopolous（医生）

47 Elm Terrace

London N14

4 December, 2017

Consultant Physician

Hammersmith Hospital

Du Cane Road

London W12

Dear Dr,

Re: Charles Oxley 26, 3, 42 (m) 42 Liverpool Way N14

This man has complained backache on and off for two years. Recently he has also complained of vague discomfort in the left side of his abdomen. This is not related to food intake. Micturition and bowels were normal. OE showed limitation of movements of spine. Abdomen NAD. Perhaps the abdomen pain originates in the spinal column and I should appreciate your opinion of him.

Yours sincerely,

Michael Apostopolous (Dr.)

2. 颅内出血(Intracranial hemorrhage)

亲爱的 ×××先生:

俞先生,35 岁,于 9 月 7 日晚被送到我院。据病史,他在 2017 年 9 月 7 日下午 2 时半进行爆破时被一根重木头击中头部。当时清醒,但在前往潘古玛医院途中失去知觉。下午 5 时到达该医院,其前约 15 分钟,失去知觉。在该医院,玛丽·梅哈大夫给他检查时,发现他神志完全不清,右颞部有湿软肿胀块,该侧瞳孔固定不动且扩大,巴宾斯基征阳性,右侧眼底模糊。诊断为颅内出血,并建议将患者转至尼克松纪念医院。

2017 年 9 月 7 日下午 11 时许,我在尼克松纪念医院见到患者,发现他神志不清,右侧瞳孔固定而扩大。头颅 X 线透视显示右侧顶骨有长线样骨折。因手术室的某些问题,直到 9 月 8 日上午才进行手术。术中恰在右侧顶骨骨折处发现硬膜外血肿,挖出许多血凝块,发现脑明显向内移位,挖出血凝块后,发现动脉血自上方和前方流出。我们不能确定出血的血管。鉴于工作条件的限制,我决定放置引流条止血。

患者于 9 月 8 日静脉注射氨苄西林 500mg,每 6 小时 1 次,手术后静脉注射地塞米松 4mg,每 4 小时 1 次。

手术后,患者一般情况仅稍好转,神志仍完全不清,第2天拆除引流条后,如无严重脑水肿,预计患者情况也许进一步改善。我没理由怀疑手术时还有硬膜下血肿。

脉搏120次/分,血压稳定,约120/70mmHg(16/9kPa,1mmHg=0.133kPa),因处理这样的患者会使我院资源过于紧张,我们亦不能足以应付手术后重大并发症,故欲将其转至贵院。

谢谢您接收该患者。

您忠诚的

J. K. 欧苏·安沙

Nixon Memorial Hospital

Southern Province

September 9, 2017

The team leader of the Chinese Medical Team

Rotifunk Hospital

Southern Province

Dear Sir,

Mr. Yu. a 35-year-old patient, was referred to our hospital in the night of September 7th. According to his history, he was struck on the head by a heavy log at 2:30 p.m. on September 7, 2017, while blasting. He was conscious for some time but on his way to Panguma Hospital he became unconscious. He arrived at Panguma Hospital at 5:00 p.m. and had been unconscious about fifteen minutes before arrival at the hospital. On examination at Panguma by Dr. Mary Maher, he was found to be fully unconscious, to have boggy swelling of the right temple with a fixed dilated right pupil and positive Babinski sign. The right fundus was blurred. She made a diagnosis of intracranial hemorrhage and advised the patient's transfer to Nixon

Memorial Hospital.

I saw the patient at Nixon Memorial Hospital around 11:00 p.m. September 7, 2017 and I found him unconscious and with a fixed dilated right pupil. X-rays of his skull showed a long linear fracture of the right parietal bone. Owing to some theatre problems, we could not start the operation until the morning of the eighth of September. At the operation we found an extra-dural haematoma just where the right parietal fracture is. We evacuated a lot of blood clot and found the brain very much displaced inwards. After evacuating the clot, we could see arterial bleeding from above in front. We could not locate the bleeding vessels and I decided to pack in order to arrest the bleeding in view of the difficult conditions under which we were working.

The patient was put on IV Ampicinin 500mg. 6-hourly on September 8. He has also been put on Dexamethason 4mg, 4-hourly since after the operation.

The patient's general condition has improved only very slightly but he has remained fully unconscious since after the operation. I expect that his condition may improve further when I remove the pack tomorrow provided he has no serious cerebral edema. I had no cause to suspect additional sub-dural haematoma at the operation.

The pulse is 120/min. B.P. is stable around 120/70mmHg (16/9kPa). I like to transfer him to you since his management will overstretch the resources of this hospital and we cannot adequately cope with major postoperative complications. Thank you for taking him over.

Sincerely yours,

(Signature)

J.K. Owusu-Ansah

3. 精神混乱（Mental aberration）

亲爱的肯诺思：

（有关 M Calthorpe 夫人的病历，5，10，1957，4 Judd Street Birmingham）

您如能为上述病人安排一次会诊我将非常感激。望您能尽快为她诊病，因为近期她将返回格拉斯哥。谨此表示感谢！

正如您看到的她的病历记录所及，她于 2005 年 9 月因小肠梗阻而入院治疗，其原因系胆囊切除术、阑尾切除术和剖腹产所致的肠粘连。发病急性期，其女儿及医生们注意到病人有精神混乱现象，但此现象随着病情的好转而消失。去年春天，我见到她时，她还有左腹痛，后来证实是由于憩室病引起的，但以后没有再犯病。她回到格拉斯哥就单独生活，一个月前她来看女儿时，又发现越来越健忘，傍晚疲劳时尤为明显。她醒的很早，总是早上五点半醒来，七点半起床。她否认自己有精神抑郁的表现，而且对自己的症状不像其女儿那样重视。她能读书，而且读完一页后能记住该页的内容。但她往往将日子搞错，如将 2 月 27 日周二说成是 2017 年 2 月 24 日。我想补充一点的是，几年来她一直用甲状腺素（100mcg），最近检查游离 T_3 正常；血红蛋白、白细胞计数、尿素、电解质、钙和肝功能亦均正常。

我想她大概认为其表现是由于自己 60 岁高龄所致。但鉴于她的间断性症状，故特请您高诊。

多谢。

您的忠实的

乔治·韦伯斯特 (Dr)

47 Elm Terrace
London N14
4 December, 2017

Consultant Physician
Hammersmith Hospital
Du Cane Road
London W12

Dear Kenneth,

Mrs. M Cathorpe 5, 10, 1957, 4 Judd Street, Birmingham

I should be grateful if you would arrange an appointment for the above patient. She is shortly returning to Glasgow so I would be grateful if you could see her fairly soon.

As you will see from her notes, she was admitted in December 2005 with small bowel obstruction, attributed to adhesions from a previous cholecystectomy, appendicectomy and Caesarian section. At the time of this acute illness, she was noted by her daughter and the doctors to be confused, but this seemed to resolve as she improved. I saw her last Spring when she had left–sided pain in the abdomen, which was probably related to the diverticular disease we subsequently demonstrated and this has not been a problem any more. She returned to an independent existence in Glasgow but when she came to visit her daughter a month ago was noted again to be increasingly forgetful. This seemed to be worse when tired in the evenings. She has always woken earlyat 5 am, rising at 7:30 a.m. She denies depression, and does not seem as concerned by her symptoms as her daughter. She is able to read and can remember the contents of the page when she gets to the end of it. However, she did get the date wrong on Tuesday, 27th February when she said it was 24th February 2017. I should add that she has been on thyroxine 100mcg for some years and that her free T_3, was checked and found to be normal recently, as was her haemoglobin, white count, urea, electrolytes, calcium and liver function tests.

I think she probably accepts that is a manifestation of her age of 60, but the intermittent nature of her symptoms prompted me to suggest that she should consult you.

With many thanks,

Yours sincerely,

George Webster (Dr)

第九节　会诊医生给开业大夫的信
（Letter to GP from consultant）

医院的医生看过病人后必须给开业医生回信,写信的内容通常包括:

（1）病人的姓名、年龄、性别、住址。

（2）病人表现的症状。

（3）从病历中所获得的进一步情况。

（4）从检查身体中获得的新发现。

（5）需要做的检验。

（6）暂时性的或确切的诊断。

（7）所需的治疗:

a. 无需治疗。

b. 内科治疗:所用药物强度、剂量、数量。

c. 住院治疗。

d. 外科治疗。

e. 精神病学治疗。

（8）预后。

（9）已给予病人的指导。

（10）保持继续联系以及将来的安排。

1. 末端回肠病变（Terminal ileal disease）

亲爱的医生：

T Baxter 先生，出生日期：1986 年 10 月 3 日，住址：10 Victoria Crescent, Cheltenham。

您的病人几次未能如约前来，这周来找我看病，他于三周前完成了回结肠部位的克罗恩病的类固醇治疗。目前病人体重增长了 8.6kg，自认为已恢复正常且食欲很好，但偶有腹痛，自述前几周他一直感冒。现在他已停用所有药物。他做过 18 个月的油漆工，现正在找工作。

查体除右下腹有轻微触痛外，未发现肿块，未发现其他任何明显异常体征。

最近的检查显示该病人血红蛋白正常，白细胞数轻度增高至 13.3（10.01 嗜中性细胞）；红细胞沉降率增至 30（1~15）；白蛋白由治疗前的 16 增至 36；碱性磷酸酶由 205 降至 124（30~100）。其余生化化验均正常。最近小肠灌肠检查确诊末端回肠病变，但在更高部位未见异常。

我曾向他及陪伴他的母亲强调定期随访的重要性。

我将于 2 个月后再看他。

您的忠诚的

会诊内科医生亨利·西蒙斯

Department of Medical

St Luke's Hospital

Cheltenham

4 May, 2017

Dr. R Graves

16 Fosseway

Cheltenham

Dear Doctor,

Mr. T Baxter 3, 10, 86(m), 10 Victoria Crescent, Cheltenham

After failing to keep several follow–up appointments, your patient came to see me this week, having finished the steroids for his ileocolonic Crohn's disease 3 weeks ago. He has regained 8.6 kg in weight and says he is now back to normal and eating well. He still gets occasional abdominal pain, and says he has had a persistent cold for the last few weeks. He is off all medication, and looking for a job after 18 months as a painter.

I could not find any significant signs on examination, apart from slight tenderness in the right lower quadrant but no mass was palpable.

His recent investigations show normal haemoglobin, with a slightly raised white count of 13.3 (10.01 neutrophils), and an ESR of 30 (1–15). His albumin has risen from the pre–treatment level of 16 to 36, and his alk. phos. has fallen from 205 to 124 (30–100). The rest of his biochemical tests are normal. The recent small bowel enema confirmed the terminal ileal disease but did not show any abnormalities higher up.

I have emphasized to him and his mother, who accompanied him, the importance of regular follow–up.

I will see him again in 2 months' time.

Yours sincerely,

Henry Simmons

Consultant Physician

2. 吸烟者支气管炎（Smoker's bronchitis）

尊敬的沃克尔医生：

患者：沙米尔·李斯特，男性，1960 年 7 月 2 日出生，家住新桥 Terrace Park 32 号。

　　我同意你的意见，即患者的疾病是吸烟者支气管炎伴气道堵塞。他的呼出气峰流速并非我曾想象的那样坏，是 245，当然总的是降低了。X 线胸片显示有轻度尘肺改变，依我看没有充足理由将其划入尘肺组内。当然，对他向尘肺医疗小组提出申请一事我没有反对意见。

　　只要李斯特先生继续吸烟，其呼吸功能障碍就会缓慢加重。若使用舒喘灵雾化吸入剂治疗，可助其在清晨排痰。我向他解释了正确的使用剂量，即每次治疗时仅喷一下，必要时可重复一次，但在 3 小时内使用量不能多于两下。如您愿让患者在今后复诊，请事先告知我们。

你最忠实的
约翰·汉密尔顿（顾问医师）

Chest Hospital
New-bridge
20 March, 2017

Dr. Robert Walker

4 St Bede's Road

New-bridge

Dear Dr. Walker,

　　Samuel Lister (M), who was born on 2nd, July, 1960, 32 Park Terrace New-bridge

　　Yes, I agree with you that the patient's trouble is smoker's bronchitis with airways obstruction. His peak expiratory flow rate is not as bad as I thought it would be, 245, but of course it is grossly reduced. The chest X-ray film shows minimal dust change which, in my opinion, is not sufficient to qualify him as a case of pneumoconiosis. There is, of course, no objection to his putting in a claim.

　　Mr. Lister can expect slow deterioration in his breathing as long as he continues smoking. It may help him to clear his chest in the morning if he has a salbutamol inhaler. I have explained to him the correct dose is one puff, repeated if necessary, and then no more for at least three hours. Please let us know if you would like him to be seen again in the future.

Yours sincerely,

John Hamilton

Consultant Physician

3. 胃—食道反流（Gastro-esophageal reflex）

亲爱的 Owen 医生：

　　姓名：Elena Cooper（女），出生日期：1960 年 7 月 4 日；住址：NW5 区 Downside Terrace，3 号。

　　感谢您来信把这位病人介绍给我。在过去的 5 周，她感到在饭后两小时或弯腰时出现反胃，烧心和呃逆。热茶导致烧灼感。她正发胖。3 天的宗教斋戒后，她就吃鱼和炸薯片。这似乎使症状加重。以往，在大吃大喝后也有较轻的类似症状。她的母亲、姐姐和哥哥有明显的胆结石家族史。

　　经检查无明显异常。我认为可能是伴有食道裂孔疝的胃 – 食道反流。我已经安排她做钡餐和腹部超声检查，同时，在我下次给她看病以前，我已给她开了胃复安和小苏打，并对她的饮食习惯提出建议。

你的真诚的

Dand Layfon

顾问医生

Whittington Hospital
Highgate Hill
London N19
15 February, 2017

Dr. Peter Owen
6 Kentish Town Road
London NW5

Dear Dr. Owen

Elena Cooper (F), who was born on 4th, July, 1960, and lived in 3 Downside Terrace NW5.

Thank you for your letter about this patient. For the past five weeks she has noticed regurgitation, heartburn and belching coming on two hours after food or on bending. Hot tea burns her. She is gaining weight. Her symptoms seem to have been precipitated by a three day religious fast terminated by fish and chips! She has had milder similar symptoms in the past after large meals. There is a strong family history of gallstones in her mother, sister and brother.

On examination there were no significant abnormalities. I think this is gastro–esophageal reflux with a possible hiatus hernia. I have ordered a barium meal and an abdominal ultrasound. I have meanwhile given her a supply of Maxolon and Sodium bicarbonate until I next see her and have advised her about her eating habits.

Yours sincerely,
David Layton
Consultant Physician

4. 泌尿系感染（Urinary infections）

亲爱的 Popplewell 医生：

　　姓名：Pamela Harvey，女，1985 年 6 月 7 日生，住址：Park Close N6。

　　感谢你提供给我一个有趣的病例。这个病人自结婚 6 年以来，大约每 4 个月发生一次泌尿系感染，然而这些感染与性交没有明显的关系，也没有什么其他促发因素。每次发作经治疗很快好转，并且没有迹象证明存在永久的肾损伤。她母亲和姐姐都有类似的症状，这是个很有趣的家族史。她母亲长期依靠药物预防，一旦停药就旧病复发。

　　通过查体及直肠检查，除了乙状结肠有轻度触痛外，没有发现任何明显的体征。为了排除其他潜在病因，我给她预约一个静脉肾盂造影和有关的其他检查。

　　如果没有什么发现，建议她按她母亲的方法长期用药物预防。

您的真诚的

David Layton

内科会诊医生

Whittington Hospital

Highgate Hill

London N19

5 January 2017

Dr. S Popplewell

10 York Rise

London N6

Dear Dr Popplewell,

　　Pamela Harvey (F), who was born on 7th, Jun, 1985, and lived in 53 Park Close N6.

Thank you for referring this patient who gives an interesting history of frequent urinary infections occurring about every 4 months since married 6 years ago. However, there is no clear–cut relation to intercourse nor is there any other precipitating factor. Each attack seems to respond rapidly to treatment and there is nothing to suggest permanent renal damage. This is an interesting family history with her mother and sister having similar symptoms. Her mother is on long–term prophylaxic and she has relapses if she ever stops taking the tablets.

I could not find any significant signs on general and rectal examination apart from slight tenderness over the sigmoid colon. I have ordered IVP and other relevant investigations to exclude any underlying cause.

Should nothing be found, it might be advisable to treat her in the same way as her mother with long–term chemoprophylaxis.

Yours sincerely,
David Layton
Consultant Physician

5. 精神分裂症（Schizophrenia）

尊敬的 Hornby 医生：

Maureen Cleaver (F) 15, 10, 1986, 35 Lillie Road SW6。

非常感谢您把茂琳 – 克列渥介绍给我们。我同意您的看法，她好像有精神分裂症样疾病的某些早期症状。我已在我们地区总医院为她安排了一张病床。我当然会在体格和精神两方面对她进行全面的观察。

如您所知，她认为她怀了双胞胎。她对现在仍有月经并不感到迷惑不解。她自诉听到有人说："茂琳是上帝的母亲！她已被特别地选择上了"，等等。她提到与一位同事不睦，这位同事曾建议她去找你看病。

她母亲是 60 岁的寡妇，已退休，住在伯明翰。她的父亲于 7 个月前故去了。她是唯一的一个孩子。她家庭气氛非常冷漠。我还未能证实有无精神病家族史。我请求与她母亲讨论她的问题，但她母亲未做答复。

茂琳出生和成长发育显然正常。她常常不出校门，避免交际，不参加运动和其他社会活动。她的学习成绩中等，她当前的工作是秘书，这是她第一次工作。12 岁月经初潮，无性生活经历，无精神病史，也无扰乱社会的行为。无滥用药物及酗酒的历史。

她系未经产妇，体格良好。表现非常躁动，甚至每次不能静坐 1~2 分钟以上的时间。虽然她偶然心烦意乱，但她说话有逻辑性。面部表情茫然，有时有些困惑，但无惊恐和压抑的表现。她说她感到沮丧并总是哭叫。她滔滔不绝地讲述那些我所提及的不正常的经历和信念，与其他具有迫害性质的想法交织在一起。她有充分定向能力，近期和远期回忆完好。对我让她所做的任何仿效性和建设性试验没有任何困难。

现在谈长期治疗和预后问题还为时过早。很清楚，她的病是功能性的。是一次具有某些压抑特征的急性发作。我们渴望她能迅速恢复并返回工作岗位。但是，她与社会的普遍隔离提示她在发病前已有病态人格，并且甚至可能是一种病变恶化过程中更隐性的发作。这只有时间才能搞清楚。有关她的病情变化，我一定与您保持联系，随时向您介绍。如果她可能及早出院的话，我愿与您讨论她的情况。

您的忠诚的
精神病科会诊医生
卡利福德·单盟德

Institute of Psychiatry
De Crespigny Park
London SE5 BAF
3 March, 2017

Dr. G Hornby
102 Fulham Road
SW6

Dear Doctor Hornby,

Maureen Cleaver (F), who was born on 15th, Oct. 1986, and lived in 35 Lillie Road SW6.

Thank you very much for referring Maureen Cleaver to us. I agree with you that she does seem to be suffering from some of the initial symptoms of a schizophrenia–like illness. I have arranged for her to be admitted to one of our beds in the district general hospital. We will of course fully investigate her both physically and psychologically.

As you know she believes that she is pregnant with twins. She is not puzzled by the fact that she is also menstruating at present. She describes hearing voices which have said: 'Maureen is the mother of God. She has been specially chosen', etc. She mentioned that she was unwell to a colleague at work who suggested that she see you.

Her mother is a 60–year–old retired widow living in Birmingham and her father died seven months ago. She was an only child and the family atmosphere was rather cold. I have been unable to establish whether there is any family history of mental illness. Her mother has not replied to my requests to discuss Maureen's problems with her.

Maureen apparently had a normal birth and development.

She kept to herself at school and avoided sporting and other social occasions. She had an average level of academic performance and is currently in her first job as a secretary. Her menarche was at 12 years and she has had no sexual experiences. There is no previous medical or psychiatric history nor has there been any anti-social behaviour and she does not abuse drugs or alcohol.

She is physically well and nulliparous. She was very restless and could not sit still for more than a minute or two at a time. Her speech was logical though occasionally she became distracted. Her expression was blank and occasionally somewhat perplexed, but not frightened or depressed. She said that she had been feeling low-spirited and crying and she freely described the abnormal experiences and beliefs which I have mentioned, together with others of a more persecutory nature. She was fully orientated, had excellent short and long-term recall and had no difficult with any of the copying and constructional tests that I asked her to do.

It is still too early to talk about long-term management and prognosis. Her illness is clearly functional, with an acute onset with some depressive features and one hopes that she will be rapidly restored and able to return to work. However, her general social isolation suggests a poor premorbid personality and even the possibility of a more insidious onset of a deteriorating process, which only time can make clear. I shall certainly keep you informed about her progress and, if an early discharge seems possible, I would like to discuss her with you.

Yours sincerely,
Clifford Drummond
Consultant Psychiatrist

6. 二尖瓣黏液变性（Myxomatous degeneration of mitral valve）

尊敬的 Crisp 医生：

R Waites (M) 4, 6, 71, 15 Faber Road Newcastle upon Tyne。

感谢您告诉我去看这位男性患者以及有关他的很有帮助的来信。他胸部不适的病史已有八个月之久，而且越来越严重。虽然胸部不适通常发生在运动时，但吃饭及性交后也有发生。胸部有时伴有心悸，但不伴有气短。

既往在儿童时期患过肺炎，也做过阑尾炎切除术。我注意到，他抽烟很多，每周喝一瓶威士忌酒。无冠状动脉性心脏病家族史。

检查：血压正常，无心力衰竭征象，脉搏规律正常，80 次 /min。听诊心尖搏动正常，心音正常，但有晚期收缩期杂音，最强点在心尖部，向胸骨右缘放散。其余体检正常。无感染性心内膜炎和肝病的征象。胸部 X 线检查正常。休息时心电图除显示在下壁组导联有非特异性 ST 段和 T 波改变外，其他方面均正常。超声心动图显示左室腔、主动脉和左心房均正常。二尖瓣运动的类型提示瓣膜脱垂。左心室壁运动非常正常。

我想此男病人可能患有二尖瓣黏液变性，此种变性导致二尖瓣反流。这在血液动力学方面并无重要意义。应鼓励他完全正常地生活。唯一需要注意的是在做任何有脓毒性感染倾向的手术操作时需用抗菌素进行保护性预防。

您的忠诚的
会诊内科医师、心脏病学家
史蒂文医学博士

Cardiology Department
Royal Victoria Infirmary
Newcastle upon Tyne
7 December, 2016

Dr Crisp
Abbotts Health Centre
14 Crispin Way
Newcastle upon Tyne

Dear Dr. Drisp,

R Waites (M), who was born on 4th, June, 71, and lived in 15 Faber Road Newcastle upon Tyne.

Thank you for asking me to see this man and for your helpful letter about him. He gives a history of chest discomfort which has been present for 8 months and is getting progressively worse. Although the chest discomfort usually occurs with exercise it can occur after eating and after sexual intercourse. The pain is sometimes associated with palpitation but he has not noticed any associated shortness of breath.

In the past he had pneumonia as a child and had also had an appendicectomy. I note that he smokes quite heavily and drinks a bottle of whisky per week. There is no family history of coronary artery disease.

On examination he is normotensive and there is no evidence of heart failure. His pulse is 80, regular and of normal character. His apex beat is normal on auscultation. He has normal heart sounds but has a late systolic murmur, maximal at the apex. It radiates to the left sternal edge. The remainder of the physical examination is normal and there are no stigmata of infective endocarditis or of liver disease. His investigations show a normal chest X-ray. His resting ECG shows some non-specific ST segment and T-wave changes in the inferior leads. It is otherwise normal. His echocardiogram shows a normal left ventricular cavity, normal aorta and left atrium. The pattern movement of the mitral valve suggests a prolapse of the valve. The left ventricular wall movements are quite normal.

I think it is likely that this man has a myxomatous degeneration of his mitral valve which is causing mitral regurgitation. This is of no haemodynamic importance and he should be encouraged to lead an entirely normal life. The only precaution he needs is for antibiotic cover for any potentially septic procedures.

Yours sincerely,
Dr P Stevens MD FRCP
Consultant Physician & Cardiologist

第十节　贺信（Congratulation）

贺信是用来表示一种礼仪的信函。人们在祝贺某人时常用一种表示祝愿、希望的贺词来表示自己的心情。单位之间，亲朋之间在重要事件面前经常互相慰勉、庆贺。贺信就是在这种情况下对某人或某事表示祝贺的文章。

贺信是特别容易写的，写起来也特别使人愉快，因为人们都乐于把别人的喜事看作是自己的喜事，这种信是鼓舞人心的书信，可以尽情地发挥。

1. 祝贺任院长（Congratulation on one's election to deanship）

亲爱的 ××× 博士：

获悉您当选为 ×× 大学 ×× 学院院长，真令人高兴万分。我深信对这种荣誉您当之无愧。过去几年，您那样勤奋地工作，今得此回报，自是理所当然。

我再一次对您荣升表示衷心祝贺。

祝你工作顺利，硕果累累。

您的忠诚的

×××

Dear Dr. ...,

Great was my delight when I learned of your election to the deanship of the ... Branch at the University of ... . I'm sure this honour is much deserved. You have worked so deligent during the last few years that is no wonder that you are reaping your rewards.

Once again, I express my congratulations on your promotion.

May success crown your every endeavor.

Yours devoted friend,

(Sinature)

...

2. 祝贺获博士学位（Congratulation on one's attainment of the Ph. D. ）

亲爱的 ×××：

获悉你已取得 ×× 大学博士学位，非常高兴。请接受我的热烈祝贺。我相信，你该多么自豪、幸福啊！你这么年轻就在学业上取得了如此卓著成绩，实在令人钦佩。我真羡慕你前程远大。我一直怀着十分敬佩的心情注视着你的进步。你不仅学习成绩优秀，而且积极参加许多社会活动。从每一个方面来说，你都正稳步而迅速地成长为一个全面发展的学者。

从你在大学和研究生院的优异成绩来看，我完全相信，今后不管做什么工作，你都会同样顺利成功。

你今后有什么打算？你是打算从事某个方面的科研工作，

利用你的科学知识造福于国家和人民,还是打算从事教学工作?不管你有什么打算,我都乐于知道。

您的真诚的

×××

Dear …,

    I was delightful to learn that you had received your Doctor's degree from … University. Accept my congratulations. I am sure that you are proud and happy. To have reached this milestone in your scholarship at such a young age is simply great. I really envy you the opportunities ahead of you. I have watched your progress with great admiration. You are not only excellent in academics, but also very active in many social activities. In every respect, you are steadily and quickly maturing into a well-rounded scholar.

    Judging by your excellent records both at the university and graduate school, I am confident that you will be equally successful in whatever career you pursue.

    What are your plans? Do you intend to work in some field of scientific research and apply your knowledge of science to bringing benefit to the country and the people, or do you intend to teach? Whatever your intentions are, I shall enjoy hearing about them.

Sincerely yours,

(Signature)

…

3. 祝贺获科技发明奖(Congratulation on one's wining an award of scientific invention)

亲爱的 × × × 先生:

    我怀着极其喜悦的心情,衷心祝贺您由于在应用化学领域从事创造性的工作而获得一等发明奖。我知道，这是您多年艰苦努力和进行无数次实验的成果。我已经听人说过您在研究方面的卓越成就。大家都说，您获此殊荣当之无愧。这表明，您的学术造诣和献身科学事业的精神，已赢得公认。我相信，这只是您获得的第一个荣誉，今后会享有更多的荣誉。您的同事有足够理由为您骄傲，您自己也完全有理由引以自豪。作为您的朋友，我非常高兴地分享您的荣誉和骄傲。

祝您在今后的事业中取得更大的成绩。

您的真诚的

×××

Dear Mr. ...,

It is with the greatest pleasure that I offer you my sincerest congratulations on your wining the first-class science award for your creative work in the field of applied chemistry. I know that it followed many years of hard work and numerous experiments on your part. I have heard of your excellent achievements in studies. Everybody says that you are worthy of the award. This shows that your outstanding scholarly attainments and whole-hearted devotion to science have been given public recognition. I am sure that this is just the first of the many honours to be bestowed upon you. Your colleagues have good reason to be proud of you, and you have every reason to be proud of yourself. As your friend, I share your honour with pride.

You have my best wishes for great success in all that you undertake.

Sincerely yours,

(Signature)

...

4. 祝贺生日（Congratulation on one's birthday）

亲爱的 ×××:

祝贺你这个幸福的时刻。祝你今年和以后的生日美满快乐。

您的真诚的

×××

Dear ...,

Congratulations on this happy day. The best of all good things for this birthday and for many more.

Sincerely yours,

(Signature)

...

5. 祝贺毕业（Congratulation on one's graduation）

亲爱的 ×××:

正因为我们之间关系密切友好的缘故吧,你毕业的消息对我来说真是件特大喜讯。在此,谨向你表示我最衷心的祝贺和最美好的祝愿。

希望你满怀信心的继续学习,发挥你具有的泉涌般的聪明才智。我愿在此补充一句,"毕业"这个词没有结束的含义,相反,按照韦氏大词典所说,"毕业"一词的基本含义是通过一个阶段,再逐步地进取。

祝你健康、幸福,在你的拼搏中取得卓著的成就。

您的真诚的

×××

Dear …,

　　Your graduation means a great deal to me particularly because of my close friendship with you. I extend my best wishes and congratulations to you.

　　I hope that you will find it possible to continue your studies and develop the talents and skills with which you are abundantly of finality to the word "graduation". On the contrary, according to Webster's Collegiate Dictionary, the basic definition of the word "graduate" is to pass by degree, to change gradually.

　　May you have health, happiness and outstanding success in all your ventures.

Sincerely,

(Signature)

…

6. 祝贺获硕士学位（Congratulation on one's Master degree）

亲爱的×××：

　　祝贺你获得硕士学位,这是令人美慕的成绩。希望你感到自豪和幸福,因为你是当之无愧的。

　　我也确信并希望毕业典礼将真正成为一个新开端,而成功之路就在你眼前。

　　祝你的事业一帆风顺,并希望你尽享为事业奋斗的愉快和幸福。

您的真诚的

×　×　×

Dear ...,

    Congratulations! Earning your Master degree is an achievement of note, and I hope you are feeling proud and happy—as you deserve.

    I am hopeful and confident, too, that the graduation ceremonies will really be a "Commencement" and that satisfying and rewarding experiences await you.

    I wish you well in all your undertaking and hope that you will find your career a source of great joy and happiness.

Sincerely,

(Signature)

...

7. 祝贺晋升（Congratulation on one's promotion）

亲爱的 ×××：

    获悉你晋升为生物化学系副教授，我很高兴并表示祝贺。熟悉你的人都知道这次晋升是你近五年来努力的结果。你一定会感到自豪，我认为你是当之无愧的。像你这样的能力难以埋没良久。相信这次晋升只是你事业腾飞的奠基石。盼望听到你下次荣升的消息。

    再次表示祝贺，并对你的前程致以最美好的祝愿。

您的真诚的

×××

Dear ...,

    I am delighted to hear of your promotion to Associate Professor in the Biochemistry Department. Congratulation! All of us who know you, know that your promotion is due to the hard work you have done for last five years. You must be proud of yourself and I think that you have every reason to be. Ability such as yours can't be hidden for long, I am sure this promotion is just steppingstone to even greater things. I look forward to hearing of your next success.

　　With many congratulations and my best wishes for the future,

Sincerely yours,

(Signature)

…

8. 祝贺获奖（Congratulating on one's prize）

亲爱的 ×××：

　　高兴地获悉你在比赛中获得二等奖。凭心而论,你在全州当名列前茅。

　　你的所有朋友都在为你自豪。

你的真诚的

×××

Dear …,

　　I was delighted to hear that you won second prize in the contest. It must feel good to know that you rank among the best in the state.

　　All of your friends are proud of you.

Cordially,

…

9. 祝贺获名誉教授称号（Congratulation on one's being conferred Honourary Professorship）

亲爱的 ××× 先生：

　　获悉您被授予 ×× 大学名誉教授,我们 ×× 医学院的全体教职工都非常高兴,并向您表示衷心的祝贺。我知道只有您才配享此殊荣。

请接受我最美好的祝愿。

您的真诚的

×××

Dear Mr. …,

All of us at … Medical College take great pleasure in sending congratulations to you upon having an Honourary Professorship conferred by … University. I know no one who deserves it more than you.

Our very best wishes to you.

Sincerely,

(Signature)

…

10. 祝贺圣诞节（Congratulation on Christmas）

亲爱的 ×××：

在此谨向你和我院在美国的同事们祝圣诞快乐和新年愉快!

请把这个祝愿转达给所有其他人。

顺致最诚挚的谢意!

您的真诚的

×××

Dear …,

This is to wish you and our colleagues of our college in America a Merry Christmas and a Happy New Year.

Kindly pass this message on to all others.

With kindest regards to you all, we remain.

Sincerely yours,

(Signature)

…

11. 贺信参考用语

多么振奋人心的(美妙的)(令人激动的)(愉快的)消息!

What exciting (wonderful) (thrilling) (happy) news!

这是个好(重大的)(惊人的)消息,(这是我长期以来听到的最愉快的消息。)

It's good (great) (sensational) news (the most joyful news I have heard for a long time).

母亲刚才告诉我们这(重大的)(令人高兴的)消息。

Mother just told us the (momentous) (cheerful) news.

听到(得到)这个消息(得到这个通知)(在报上看到……)我很高兴(振奋)(惊喜)。

I was delighted (thrilled) (pleasantly) to hear (to receive) the news (to receive the announcement) (to read in the newspaper) …

好了,你终于完成了(去结婚了)(晋升了)!

So you've done it (gone and got married) (been promoted)!

好,你和汤姆终于订婚了!

So you and Tom are engaged!

祝贺你……

I congratulate you …

祝贺……

Congratulations on …

热烈地(衷心地)祝贺……

Warm (Sincere) congratulations ...

我们如此兴奋地（高兴地）（激动地）获悉（从这一消息中获悉）……

We were so excited (delighted) (thrilled) to hear (by the news) ...

恭贺您并致以良好（最良好）的祝贺。

Congratulations and all good (best) wishes!

您可能不知道我听到这消息时是多么地激动（快乐）……

You have no idea what a thrill (great pleasure) I got when I heard ···

请接受我最衷心的祝贺……

Accept my heartiest congratulations ...

请允许我向您祝贺……

Permit me to congratulate you ...

我们大家祝愿你……

Best wishes from all of us on ...

（对于）……谨致最良好的祝愿。

Our best wishes ...

（对于）……致以最良好的祝愿

Best of the best wishes ...

……我们真诚地祝愿您幸福无比。

We certainly wish you all the happiness in the world ...

祝您（俩）一切顺利。

The best of everything (to both of you).

（对于）……谨致以最诚挚的良好祝愿。

The heartiest good wishes ···

祝一切顺利（万事如意）（无比幸福）。

Loads and loads of good luck (good wishes) (happiness).

祝您无比幸运。

All the luck in the world to you.

久闻她的大名（我们渴望和她见面）。

We have heard so much about her (we are eager to meet her).

我认为您是个幸运的人。

I think you're a lucky guy.

我认为这真是了不起！

I think it's swell!

在任何一方面她都是个了不起的（漂亮的）（出色的）（非凡的）（极好的）（非常可爱的）（美丽的）姑娘。

She's a wonderful (fine) (splendid) (marvelous) (charming) (very lovely) (pretty) girl in every way.

她将成为您的出色的（美丽的）（迷人的）妻子。

She will make you a wonderful (excellent) (charming) wife.

向您（脱帽）致敬！

My hat's off to you!

我以有您而感到骄傲。

I'm proud of you.

对您的仰慕热诚，使我欣然动笔……

My enthusiasm about you prompts me to write ...

从您的出色工作中，体现出您的计划周密，工作辛勤。

The careful planning and hard work is reflected in a job well done.

众誉所归，受之无愧。

The recognition you have received is well deserved.

请允许我向您表示热烈的祝贺。

Permit me to send my enthusiastic congratulations.

任务艰巨，而您却勇于承担，赢得声誉。

It was a tough assignment, and you handled it with credit.

这是精彩的表演（巨大的胜利）（精彩的演讲）。

It was a splendid performance (great triumph) (brilliant speech).

我尤其喜欢……

I liked especially ...

这是超级的（好的）（创记录的）……

It is a superb (fine) (record) …

我佩服您的判断力（计划性）（毅力）（独创性）（成就）（办事的能力）（令人难忘的经历）。

I admire your judgment (planning) (perseverance) (ingenuity) (achivement) (capacity to get things done) (impressive record).

这是一位老友对您生日的祝词（热烈祝贺）。

Here's a word of cheer on your birthday (warm birthday greetings) from an old friend.

祝贺您并致以良好的祝愿。

Congratulations and all good wishes.

当您的一生达到这一里程碑之际，（当您的这一重要良辰，）仅表示衷心的祝贺并致以最良好的祝愿。

Hearty congratulations and all good wishes on this milestone (wonderful day) in your life.

适值您的生日，希望您知道我们都在想念您，并愿您在生活中的一切获得满意。

I want you to know that we are thinking of you on your birthday and wishing you the best of everything life has to offer.

希望这份（薄）礼能给您的生日（今后的岁月）增添一些快乐（幸福）。

I hope this (little) gift will add a bit to your enjoyment (happiness) on your birthday (during the years ahead).

出了名，实在太好了。

How does it feel to be famous!

第十一节　慰问信（Sympathy）

慰问信是向对方表示慰问的书信。亲戚或朋友发生了不愉快或不幸的事，要及时去慰问，向对方表示同情和安慰，鼓励对方克服重重困难。写这类信,感情要真挚,措辞需贴切。

1. 慰问病人(To those who are ill)

外国人给病人的慰问信,要在病情已好转或恢复健康的时候写,也可以在病人离开病床以后再写。写得好的慰问信像你亲自去探望病人一样,给人以温暖,能为病人消愁解闷,使病人乐观、轻松。

慰问信最好写一些病人喜欢的、熟悉的外界事物。如果病人爱好打高尔夫球,就告诉他最近谁打高尔夫球打了九十分;如果病人喜欢热带鱼,就可以告诉他最近看到的热带鱼展览,或报刊上的有关报道。女主人喜欢种花,也很关心她自己的孩子,在信中可以告诉她,她的花园中的花开的多么喜人,或她的孩子长得多么可爱。总之,应该写一些病人喜欢的、有趣的事情。

亲爱的科宾夫人:

听说您生了病,我非常难过。您一定要尽快地恢复健康,因为邻居们都很想念您,大家都希望您早日出院归来。

伯克先生和我祝您很快康复。

您真挚的

玛丽·T·伯克

Dear Mrs. Corbin,

I was so sorry to learn of your illness. You must hurry and get well! Everybody in the neighborhood misses you, and we're all hoping you'll be back soon.

Mr. Burke joins me in sending best wishes for your speedy recovery.

Sincerely yours,

Mary T·Burke

＊　　　＊　　　＊

亲爱的玛丽：

听说您的病体恢复的很快，不久就要出院，回到家人和朋友当中了。这是多好的消息啊，玛丽！您生了病我感到非常寂寞，自从您住进医院以后，就一直想念您。在您生病的痛苦时刻，我简直难以形容心中是多么难过。

但是，这一切都过去了。您就要和一个很健康的人一样了。昨天我在姐姐家中遇到卡里逊医生（我姐姐的小儿子得了流行性腮腺炎）……他告诉我您是他的非常满意的病人。他说您复原的情况良好，看来很快会恢复原来那样的健康和体力。

昨天我还见到了约翰，那个可怜的人自从离开了您就像一只失群的羊！他说他在一小时一小时地数着等候您回家。珍妮特和他在一起呢，过去的一年她长得多高呀！您有个可爱的女儿，玛丽，她的仪态是那样温柔妩媚，正如她的面孔生的那么美丽一样。您一定会为她感到骄傲的。

弗兰克向您表示最美好的祝愿。他要我告诉您，当他听说您迅速地恢复健康的时候，他非常高兴。保持住这个恢复的势头，玛丽，早日回来同热爱您的、想念您的人们团聚。

您亲爱的
莉莲

Dear Mary,

I hear you are making such a rapid recovery that you'll soon be out of the hospital and back with your family and friends. That's wonderful news, Mary! I've missed you so much. You've been on my mind constantly, ever since you went to the hospital. I just can't tell you how sorry I was that you had such a difficult time of it.

But all that's over now, and you'll soon be as good as new! I met Dr. Carleson at my sister's house yesterday (her little boy has the mumps) … and he tells me you are his prize patient. He says you rallied beautifully, and that from this point on you'll show steady improvement—until you have all your old health and strength back again.

I saw John yesterday, too. The poor man is like a lost sheep without you! He says he's counting the very hours until you come home. Janet was with him; my …, how she has grown in the past year! You have a lovely daughter, Mary … as gracious and charming as she is sweet to look at. You must be very proud of her.

Frank sends his best wishes, and he says to be sure and tell you how delighted he is to hear about your fine progress. Keep it up, Mary—and come home real soon to those who love and miss you.

Affectionately
Lillian

2. 慰问受伤的人（To those who have been injured）

写给受伤的人的慰问信要尽量简短，尽量中肯。信中不必查问事故是怎么发生的，是谁的过错，或有无见证人；而应该表达你听说友人受伤后的难过心情，以及希望他不久就能痊愈等等。换言之，你关心的不应该是事故的前前后后，而应该是受伤者的身体和恢复情况。

亲爱的汤姆：

知道您受到意外伤害时，我简直难以形容我心中是多么难过。您家中的人告诉我，您恢复得很好，再有十天左右就可以出院了。听说这一情况后，我心中确实感到宽慰。

在一两天内您会收到玛格丽特和我寄给您的一份小礼物，我希望您喜欢它，它能帮助您更愉快地消遣时光。

衷心祝愿您尽快地恢复健康！

您真诚的
鲍勃

Dear Tom,

I just can't tell you how sorry I was to learn of your accident. Your family tells me that you are progressing nicely, and that you'll be out of the hospital in about ten days. I'm certainly relieved to know that!

In the next day or so you'll receive a little package from Margaret and me. I hope you like it, and that will help to pass the time more pleasantly.

With every good wish for your swift recovery,

Sincerely,
Bob

*　　　*　　　*

亲爱的玛乔里：

刚才听说小皮特在一次足球比赛中受了伤，我心中十分难过。希望他的伤势不重。

我理解您现在的心情，正像几年前乔治曾使我经受的一样——记得吗？我想男孩们在成长期间，他们的母亲是难免不碰到这类事情的。

请告诉我有什么事我可以帮助您做的。也许您想在皮特伤愈之前把帕茨送到我们这里住上一两个星期。我们很乐意接受。而且我负责把他安全地送到学校，再接回家来。给我打个电话好了，玛乔，我来接他。

告诉皮特，他受了伤我很难过，希望他不久就能完全恢复健康。

您亲爱的
哈丽特

Dear Marjory,

I've just learned that young Pete was hurt in a football game. I'm ever so sorry to hear it, and I hope his injuries are not serious.

I know just how you feel because I had the same experience with George a few years ago—remember? I guess it's just something all mothers of growing boys must expect!

Please let me know if there's anything I can do to help. Perhaps you'd like to send Patsy here for a week or so, until Pete is better. We'd love to have him, and I'd see that he got to and from school safely. Just phone me, Marj—and I'll come and get him.

Tell Pete I'm sorry he was hurt, and that I hope he'll soon be fit as a fiddle again.

Affectionately,
Harriet

3. 慰问信参考用语

愿您迅速康复（迅速恢复健康）。

We hope you will have a speedy convalescence (quick recovery).

我们深信您不久就会康复。

We're sure it won't be long before you're back on your feet again.

我们向您同致热忱的问候。

We all join in sending you our heartfelt love.

谨向您表示思念之情。

I want you to know I am thinking of you.

您的朋友们都在期望您早日恢复健康（早日痊愈）（迅速康复）（早日出院）。

Your many friends are hoping for your quick return to health (early recovery) (rapid recovery) (return from the hospital).

我们都在等待着您的归来。

All of us are waiting your return.

我们期望您很快归来（数周内能非常健康）。

We expect to see you back soon (as good as new in a few weeks).

愿您迅速地、愉快地度过康复期。

We hope your convalescence will be rapid and pleasant.

愿您迅速康复（能早日起床活动）（很快恢复健康）。

We hope you will soon regain your health (be up and about) (be feeling a lot better).

第十二节　吊唁信（Condolence）

在私人信件中，吊唁信是最难写的。因为难写，很多人宁肯用打电话、送吊唁明信片或鲜花等形式来表示哀悼，以避免写这种书信。

然而，吊唁信也可能是最有意义、最使人感激的书信。因为这种信常常能使友人得到安慰。对于那些深受打击和伤害的人，一封写得好的吊唁信，就像伸出的友谊之手，给人以温暖、信念和勇气。

写吊唁信时态度要真诚，措辞要严谨，不能滥用华丽的辞藻，也不要写得过长，因为这种时刻不是多说话的时候。在这种信中，不宜询问生病和死亡的细节，也不宜引用安慰人们的典故；尤其应避免触及病痛的根源，以防止收信人的悲伤再次爆发或加深。

在吊唁中,切忌写上像"She was too young to die!"或"Your life will be desolate without him!"一类的话。写上这类不关痛痒的话,倒不如根本不写为好。

如果你真正被一位友人的不幸所感动,确实感受到他的痛苦,深深体会到他的悲伤,在这种心情下写出一封好的吊唁信也不是十分困难的。只要笔下流露出真挚的哀悼之情,你的信就会使人倍感亲切。

下面的几封信是有代表性的,目的在于提供一些模式,帮助你写好吊唁信。

1. 讣告（Obituary notice）

讣告是一种报丧文书。某人逝世后,家属、工作单位或治丧委员会发出讣告,使死者的亲友知道事情的经过。一般写上死者的姓名、身份、职务、逝世的原因、日期、地点等。

*　　　*　　　*

××医学院院长×××教授因患肺癌,医治无效,于2017年12月25日9时28分在北京逝世,享年80岁。

×教授是一位知识渊博、受人尊敬的教育家。他把毕生精力无私地献给了医学教育事业,献给了人民和国家。他极其热情地向学生传授他的丰富知识。他的逝世使我们失去了一位尊敬的朋友和良师,对此我们感到万分悲痛。

兹定于12月28日举行遗体告别仪式,12月29日举行追悼会。凡献花圈、挽联者,请置于学校礼堂前厅。

×××教授治丧委员会

Professor ..., President of ... Medical College, died of lung cancer at 9:28, on December 25, 2017 in Beijing at the age of 80, after failing to respond to meticulous medical treatment.

Professor … was a respected educator, with great learning. He selflessly dedicated all his energies throughout his life to the cause of education, the people, and the nation. He imparted his immense store of learning to all his students with great warmth. We are deeply grieved by this death. We have all lost a dear friend and mentor.

Final respects will be paid to his remains at a mourning ceremony on Dec. 28. A memorial service will be held on Dec. 29. Flowers, wreaths and elegiac couplets are expected to be laid in the front hall of school auditorium.

The Funeral Committee for
Late Prof. …

*　　　*　　　*

亲爱的 ×××：

我们向您沉痛地宣布，×× 医学院名誉院长、著名内科学教授、临床内分泌学家 ××× 教授，于 2017 年 12 月 25 日逝世。

我们悲痛地向他的亲密朋友、同事和有关组织通知这个不幸的消息。

您的真诚的
××× 博士
×× 医学院院长

Dear …,

We regret to inform you that Prof. …, M.D. Honorary President of … Medical College, and well-known professor of internal medicine and clinical endocrinologist, passed away on December 25th 2017.

It is with great sorrow that this announcement is made to close friends, colleagues and concerned organizations.

Thank you.

Sincerely yours,

(Signature)

..., M.D.

President

... Medical College

2. 唁函（Letter of condolence）

唁函是死者亲友对死者家属或单位写的。一般包括以下3个方面：

（1）提及某人死亡，并表示沉痛的心情。

（2）提及死者的个人品格及贡献。

（3）对死者的亲人表示慰问。

*   *   *

亲爱的 ××× 夫人：

　　惊悉 ××× 教授逝世，深感悲痛。他的逝世不仅对您的家庭而且对我们学校都是一个巨大的损失。××× 教授多年来竭诚为人民服务，特别是为学生服务，是一位最优秀、最受人尊敬的老师，他也是一位著名的内科学家，在内分泌学领域做出了巨大的贡献。他为培养年轻一代和发展医学科学所做的贡献举世公认。我们失去了一位卓越的师长，再不能受益于他的才华和学识了。我们这些有幸与 ××× 教授共过事的人，都对他怀着钦佩和崇敬的心情。他对教师和学生的精心指导和热情培养，我们将永世不忘。

　　值此悲痛时刻，特致函表示深切哀悼。如需帮助，我当竭尽全力。

请向全家转致诚挚的慰问。

您的真诚的

×××

Dear Mrs. ...,

I am greatly shocked and deeply sorrowed by the passing of Prof. ... . His passing is a great loss not only to your family but also to our school. He was a most distinguished and respected teacher who had served his people and school with great devotion for many years. He is also a well-known physician who made great contributions to the field of endocrinology. His dedication to the fostering of young people and medical sciences is widely recognized. Our school will be poorer without the benefit of his wisdom and scholarship. Prof. ... inspired admiration and esteem among all of us who were privileged to work with him. We will always remember the warm and kind help that he gave to our faculty and students.

Let me assure you that I share this bitter moment with you and if there is anything that you need, I shall be entirely and heartly at your disposal.

Please convey my kindest regards and deepest condolences to your family.

Sincerely yours,

(Signature)

...

*   *   *

亲爱的 ××× 校长：

惊悉 ××× 教授逝世，深感悲痛，特此致函，深表哀悼。

我与 ××× 教授相识多年，且一向视为知己。他的溘然逝世使医学界失去了一位著名的科学家。我们这些在费城的人，均对他怀念不已。与他交往令人愉快，凡认识他的人都会深深怀念他。

请代为转达我们对 ××× 夫人和家属的关切之情。

您的真诚的
×××

Dear President ...,

We were distressed by the news that Dr. ... has died, and I am writing at once to express our deep sympathy.

I had the privilege of knowing Dr. ... for many years and always regarded him as a personal friend. By his untimely passing our medical society has lost one of its brilliant scientists. We, in Philadelphia, recall his kindness and it was always a pleasure to talk with him. He will be greatly missed by all who knew him.

Please convey our sympathy to Mrs. ... and his family.

Yours very sincerely,
(Signature)
...

3. 对于吊唁信的感谢（Thanks for a letter of condolence）

对于每一封吊唁信都应亲自写信表示感谢。

对于表示同情的吊唁信，一定要及时地回信。回信应该写得简短，能表达谢意就够了。

* * *

亲爱的 ××× 博士：

　　非常感谢您至诚至感的来信。我们的确十分悲痛。因为 ××× 大夫就是我们的一切。他从不考虑个人，而把整个生命献给了医学事业。我接触的每一个人都对他怀有爱戴和崇敬之情。总之，我们一定要面对现实，因为我们知道他希望我们这样。

　　非常感谢您提供的热诚帮助。

　　　　　　　　　　　　　　　　　您的真诚的

　　　　　　　　　　　　　　　　　×××

Dear Dr. …,

　　We all deeply appreciate your most kind letter. Our grief is indeed most bitter. Dr. … was everything to us. He never had a thought for himself, and devoted his whole life to our medical sciences. Everyone I have spoken to seems to have loved and respected him. Well, we have got to face our loss as we know he would wished us to.

　　Thank you so much for your kind offer of help.

　　　　　　　　　　　　　　　　　Yours sincerely,

　　　　　　　　　　　　　　　　　(Signature)

　　　　　　　　　　　　　　　　　…

* * *

亲爱的 ××× 博士：

　　感谢您在信中对 ××× 教授所做的高度评价，同时也感谢您寄来的唁函。的确，对 ××× 教授的逝世，我们的心情同您一样。这种不幸事件我们也不能驾驭。

　　当然，×××教授的逝世使他的家属非常悲痛，不过，他们都是很坚强的人。我们在学校礼堂为×××教授举行了一个隆重的追悼会，他的全家和朋友都出席了追悼会。

　　感谢您寄来的医疗诊断书、死亡证明书和其他遗物。我们也感谢您在处理这个不幸事件中表现出的审慎的专家风度。

您的真诚的

×××

Dear Dr. …,

　　Thank you for your very kind remarks about Professor … in your letter. Thank you also for the letter of condolences. Certainly, we felt the same way about Professor … as you. It is a very sad situation but one which is beyond our control.

　　Naturally, his death created a very grave situation for his family. They are strong people however. We held a beautiful memorial service for Prof. … here in the school auditorium. His family and friends were in attendance.

　　Thank you for sending the medical certificate, death certificate, and other personal items. We are grateful to you for the most professional and conscientious manner in which you have handled this most distressing event.

Sincerely,

(Signature)

…

4. 悼词（Memorial speech）

悼词是在死者的追悼会上发表的讲话，一般多介绍死者的身份、职务、逝世原因、时间、地点、逝世时年龄，追悼死者生前的主要经历和成就，目的在于怀念死者，激励生者，安慰家属。

*   *   *

同志们、朋友们：

　　我们怀着万分悲痛的心情悼念×××教授，他为我国的教育事业贡献了光荣的一生。

　　×××教授1923年出生于承德。他1942年考入北京协和医学院；在校期间，学习成绩优异；毕业后，曾被选派到美国哈佛医学院进修。新中国一成立，他创建了××医学院并担任第一任院长。他为我国的教育事业和医学事业贡献了毕生精力。他以治学严谨著称。除了教育工作外，他的足迹遍及中国边远地区，为解除患甲状腺肿和克汀病患者的痛苦而奔波劳碌。他坚持不懈地致力于发展医学科学，在国内外赢得高度赞誉。近年来，他一直不顾年老体弱，无私地、不知疲倦地工作着。2016年12月25日他逝世在工作岗位上。

　　我们悼念×××教授，一定要学习他全心全意为人民服务的崇高品质。×××教授一贯勤勤恳恳、任劳任怨、大公无私、谦虚谨慎、平易近人、以身作则、艰苦朴素，是我们学习的好榜样。

　　×××教授和我们永别了。我们一定要化悲痛为力量，团结一心，为实现我们可爱的社会主义祖国的四个现代化而共同奋斗。

　　×××教授，安息吧！

　　×××教授永垂不朽！

Comrades and friends,

　　It is with the deepest grief that we pay our lasting respects to the memory of Prof. ..., who died a glorious death for the educational cause of our country.

Prof. ... was born in 1923 in Chengde. In 1942, he was admitted to Peking Union Medical College where he did exceedingly well during the period of his studies. After graduation, he was sent to Harvard Medical School in the U. S. for advanced studies. Immediately after the birth of new China, he set up ... Medical College and became its first President. He dedicated himself to medical education and to the health of the nation. He was noted for his meticulous scholarship. In addition to his educational work, his footprints remain in a number of remote areas in China where his work relieved the suffering of patients with goiter and cretinism. His unceasing efforts to develop the medical sciences won him high praises in our country and in the world. In recent years, he continued to work selflessly and untiringly in spite of his advanced age and poor health. On December 25, 2016, he died at his post.

In mourning Prof. ..., we should learn from his noble qualities of serving the people. He was diligent and conscientious, hard-working and uncomplaining, indefatigable and selfless. He was modest and prudent, unassuming and easily approachable, setting a good example by his conduct and living in a plain and hardworking way. Let us mold ourselves in his image.

Prof. ... has left us, but we must turn our grief into strength, unite as one and strive to realize the four modernization goals of our beloved socialist motherland.

May you rest in peace, Prof. ... !

Eternal glory to Prof. ... !

5. 吊唁信参考用语

得知……去世的消息，我极为（万分）（非常）难过。

I was extremely (terribly) (so) sorry to hear of the death of ...

一听到（得悉）这一悲痛的消息，我们无比悲伤（沉痛）。

We have just heard (learned) with profound sorrow (regret) the sad news.

今天母亲告诉我们这一令人悲痛的消息。

Mother told us of the sad news today.

惊悉这一悲惨的消息，感到无比沉痛。

It was a profound (sad) (great) shock to hear the tragic (sad) news.

我无法表达我们是多么沉痛……

I don't have to tell you how much we regret ...

……感到无比沮丧。

It is with the greatest disappointment ...

谨向您和您一家人表示最深切的吊慰（在您悲伤的时刻我们对您深表同情）。

I want you to know how much I sympathize with you and your family (how deeply we feel for you in your sorrow).

但愿我能以什么言词或行动来安慰您（来帮助您）。

I wish there was something I could say or do to soften your grief (to help you).

我无法表达我难过的心情（我们是多么的伤心）。

I can't (must) tell you how sorry I am (how saddened we were) ...

我们万分沉痛……

We were deeply saddened ...

让我同了解和敬慕她的人（她的许多朋友）一道表示诚挚的哀悼（谨表慰问）。

May I add my sincere sympathy (small word of consolation) to that of the many who knew and admired her (to that of her countless friends).

致以我们最深切的（诚挚的）（衷心的）哀悼。

You have our deepest (sincerest) (heartfelt) sympathy.

请接受我对……的去世表示最深切的同情（诚挚的吊慰）。

Please accept my deepest sympathy (sincere condolence) on the death of …

所有认识和热爱……的人，都将分担您的悲痛。

Your sorrow is shared by everyone who knew and loved …

谨致（最）诚挚（衷心）（深切）的吊慰。

We want to offer (most) sincere (heartfelt) (deepest) sympathy.

没有任何语言能表达我对……所感到的巨大（诚挚）的悲痛。

There are no words that can express my great (sincere) (deep) sorrow at …

我知道此时此刻言语难以给您慰籍（目下没有什么言语能给你带来安慰）。

I know words are not much comfort at a time like this (there are no words that can be a comfort to you now).

如果我们能减轻您（巨大）（沉重）的悲伤该多好。

We wish it were in our power to soften your (great) (deep) sorrow.

如果有什么办法能减轻您的悲伤（沉重的悲痛）（能减轻您遭受的打击），该多好。

I wish there were some way in which we could lighten your grief (burden of sorrow) (soften the blow that has come to you).

我们向您同致诚挚的问候。

We all join in sending you our heartfelt love.

谨向您表示思念之情。

I want you to know I am thinking of you.

第十三节　英文书信通则
（The general rules of English letter）

1. 信封（Envelope）

（1）英文书信一般不将寄信人的姓名与地址写在信封的背面。大多欧美人打开信封之后即将信封弃掉，因而，如要收信人回信，应将寄信人的详细地址写在信内。

（2）收信人若为男性，正确的称谓是"某某先生"，如"J. 平特 (J Pinter) 先生"。若收信人是一位资深的外科医生，如叫罗伯特·特纳（Robert Turner），则可据此写为"罗伯特·特纳先生，皇家外科医师学会会员"。如收信人有其他学衔，亦应写明。如"彼得·卡明斯博士（Peter Cummings），皇家外科医师学会，麻醉师分会会员"和"托马斯·沃克先生 (Thomas Walke)，皇家妇产科学会会员"。

（3）收信人如有文职、军职或学术方面的荣誉称号，亦应按前列顺序书写于姓名之后。

（4）写给某学院、公司、饭店或报社等机关单位的业务信件，应写明寄给该机关的某个人，或写明某学院的院长、某公司的秘书或经理，某饭店的经理或接待员，某报纸的编辑等。

（5）写给已婚女子或遗孀的信，除非她另有其他头衔，通常称"某某太太"。

（6）写给未婚女子的信，通常称谓"某某小姐"。

（7）女士（Ms.）一词用于婚姻状态不明的女性。有些女子喜用此称呼。

（8）收信人住址按下列次序写在收信人姓名之后。

〔Ⅰ〕门牌号
〔Ⅱ〕街名　　　}写在同一行

〔Ⅲ〕城镇或乡村名
〔Ⅳ〕邮政编码　}写在同一行

〔Ⅴ〕郡

〔Ⅵ〕国家（如果信由国外邮寄）

例：Dr. John Turner MB CHB DPM

36 Pilkington Avenue

Wakefield WF2 9DG

West Yorkshire England

现代书信中姓名、地址部分一般略去标点符号。用打字机打印的书信，行首不留空格。

2. 书信（Letter）

（1）发信人详细地址写在信纸的右上方，按习惯此处不写发信人的姓名。医院等单位，常用印好地址的信笺，其地址或印在右上方或印在中间上方。

（2）日期书于地址的下方，顺序为：日、月、年（如 23 March, 2017）。私人信件可用阿拉伯数字表示，如上述日期可写作23.3.2017。

（3）商业书信中，收信人姓名、地址写在信纸左上方。

（4）给一位不相识的人写信，开头称呼应为亲爱的先生（Dear Sir），当给女士写信时（如给医院的护理主任写信时）称亲爱的夫人（Dear Madam）。

（5）如与收信人曾见过面或有一段时间通过信，信首称谓用姓氏，例如：亲爱的特纳博士（Dear Turner）。

（6）给朋友写信，信首称谓为"亲爱的"，加名如"亲爱的约翰"，"亲爱的玛丽"。给比较亲近的朋友写信，常用"我的亲爱的伊丽莎白"。

（7）如果信首写"亲爱的先生或夫人"，信的结尾应写

"Yours faithfully（你的忠实的）"。

（8）在半业务性通信中如信首用"亲爱的斯蒂尔小姐"或其他的名字，结尾应写"Yours sincerely（你的真诚的）"。

（9）"With best wishes"，"With kindest regards,"或"Yours"，通常用于写给朋友的信的结尾。

（10）"I remain your humble servant"和"Yours respectfully"已不再使用，英文信中不再使用这些辞藻华丽溢于言表的语言。业务书信更应精练、简洁。

（11）在谈及一个新的主题或事情的一个方面需分段书写时，为了使段落分明，段落的首行要留空或让行距大一些。

3. 英文书信的写作（The Writing of English Letter）

英文书信的写作，除了要掌握书写格式，善用各种称谓，注意结尾谦语，以及在形式上做到行文整齐、空白适中、字体端正外，还有不少在行文、用词方面的具体要求和习惯用法，都是值得注意的问题。现归纳如下：

（1）简洁明了，有条有理 简洁是指行文语言上的简明、通顺。包括缩短不必要的字句，剔除迂回冗长的句法，删去虚浮无当的字眼，使一封信写得尽量简短。用语浅显、易懂，不要用生僻费解的词句或一些不必要的深文奥意。比如让别人把事情做的彻底一点，可说 do it thoroughly 而不要讲 to go the whole hog. 同时要求信中所述事情必须完整，凡事有条有理，有层有次，使人读起来对前因后果，来龙去脉，一目了然。

（2）谦恭有礼，热情诚恳 所谓谦恭有礼，是指态度的谦虚与恭敬。但这不是说在措辞上加几个敬辞或讲几句客套话，而是在叙事时充分为他人着想，不要纯粹以自己为中心。这样不但给人们一种好印象，即便是推辞他人要求时，也不致失去友好的关系。此外，尽可能及时复信，如确实无法答复时，也要将原因以及何时有结果尽快函告对方，这是一种礼貌，同时也是一种办事效率高、对人热情诚恳的基本态度。

（3）删繁就简,避免冗辞　这里所说的删繁就简,可以说是继 a 项对整个行文的词句的具体要求。信以简洁为好,信文中避免一些不必要的华而不实的词句,包括一些不该使用的形容词、副词、短语等修饰词语。宁简勿繁,提高用词的效率。

（4）选词要确切,语言要规范　这是指用词和词语搭配方面要准确,合乎英语语言习惯,不要自己杜撰,拼凑或使用已过时的或不常用的行话。如:

A	B
We beg to acknowledge your esteemed favour on September 16.（过时,不常用）	We have received your letter of September 16.（9 月 16 日来信已收到。）
The writer wishes to acknowledge ...（行话）	Thank you for your letter ...（谢谢您的来信）
As per our letter ...（陈旧,不常用）	According to your letter ...（根据来信所述）

（5）内容准确,不要含含糊糊　这是说信中所谈的事情要清楚、确实,少用含糊、抽象或不具体的词句,便于收信人明了。例如要答谢别人上封来信,最好要提及那封信的具体日期、内容,不要仅写本月（instant 或 inst.）,上月（ultimo 或 ulto.）,下月（proximo 或 prox.）等字样。如:Thank you for your letter of July 5 ...（感谢你七月五日来信……）。如果收到某物后,要表示感谢,最好是要提及收到何物,而不要含糊地说。acknowledge receipt of a favour ...。

4. 英文书信的起首语和结束语(Opening and concluding sentences of English letter)

（1）起首语

I was glad to receive your letter of May 4 ...

我很高兴收到你五月四日来信……

With great delight I learn that ...

我很高兴地听说……

I have the pleasure to tell you that ...

我很愉快地告诉你……

I have just received your kind letter.

刚刚收到您的来信。

Your kind letter of Saturday arrived this morning.

星期六的来信，今早收到了。

As I have not heard of you for long, I feel anxious.

久未通信，悬念之至。

（2）结束语

I hope to hear from you soon.

希望尽快收到你的来信。

I look forward to our next meeting.

盼望下次再见。

Your kind early reply will be appreciated.

如蒙即复，不胜感激。

Won't you let us hear from you promptly?

可否即予复示？

We hope that the finished work will prove in every way satisfactory to you.

真诚地希望这项工作在各方面使你满意。

Any other particulars required I shall be pleased to give you.

如需其他详情，当欣然奉告。

The help you send is sincerely valued.

承蒙厚助，由衷感谢。

5. 几个应该注意的问题（Some Points for Attention）

首先，要及时写信或复信。这是一种礼貌，也是对对方的尊敬。看起来这似乎不算什么问题，而且我们生活中也确有不少人不愿写信或将该复的信拖的很久。但实际上，这不仅会使对方牵挂、疑虑，而且还会给对方一种不良印象，常会引起对方不满、误解，甚至使其有理由感到受了轻视或冷遇，以至伤害感情、失去友谊。所以，每当我们认为需要写信或该复信时，一定要写，而且要及时写。

再者，要选用质地优良的信纸，不要使用过于鲜艳的有色纸和有格稿纸。这不仅是为了给人一种良好印象，而且也是为了使用顺手。邀请信、感谢信以及吊唁信要使用纯白的信纸。商业信件以及一些非正规的社交信件，均可使用打字机打，其他私人信件不拘。但像社交书信中的慰问信、感谢信和一些短柬等，最好用手写体。这样会使人感到亲切、真挚。书写信件，要用钢笔，不用铅笔；使用黑色或蓝色墨水，不用红色或其他颜色的墨水。字迹要求工整，纸面要求清洁。字不管多少，应当使用整张信纸。此外，还要尽量避免拼写和语法上的错误。以上虽属一些细节，但细心注意，会使你的书信更加完美。

便条和通知（Note and notice）

便条和通知是日常生活中使用频度最高的两种文体，其特点是内容简短、格式简单，通常只有几句话，开门见山。前者一般用于熟人之间；后者则多用于上级对下级，组织对成员。

第一节　便条（Note）

便条是书信的一种形式，常用的有请假条和留言条两种。较普通书信来说，其特点是格式简单，内容简短。

由于便条大都是临时通知、询问，或在某一场合下的直接留言，谈的大多是一、两天内的事情，故写时往往是开门见山，一、两句话完事，而且格式也没有普通书信那样严格。譬如留言条，日期可以写上年、月、日，也可以写星期几或星期几上、下午，或者只写几日、几点钟也行。日期可以写在正文右上角，也可以写在末尾，即署名下一行，并没有一个严格限制。但不论采用什么形式，或者内容多么简短，一定要讲清楚这么几点，即写给谁的、什么事，谁写的以及什么时候写的。

便条尤其是留言条多用于熟悉的同事、朋友之间，往往是托人递交或者是本人临时在某一场合下的直接留言。它一般写在纸条上，格式较短柬更为简单，没有写信人地址、收信人地址、结尾语等项目，通常不用信封。用词比较通俗、口语化。譬如讲到"要告诉某人某事"可用"Just a line to tell you that"而不必用

"This is to inform you that"开头。前者是比较随便的用语,后者是比较正式的说法。再者,同样说到"延期",可用"put off",而不必用"postpone"。总之,除要注意这些区别外,还要多留意一些常用的词,留意它们的搭配和句子结构。

1. 请病假便条(Asking for sick leave)

亲爱的 ××× 先生:

很抱歉,我不能参加下午的会议。兹附上证明一张。医生说,我必须卧床休息几日后才能上班。希望我的病假不会给您造成太大的不便。

您的真诚的

×××

2016 年 12 月 20 日

Dec. 20, 2016

Dear Sir,

I am very sorry that I can not come to the meeting this afternoon. Enclosed please find a certificate from my doctor stating that I must remain in bed for a few days before returning to my office.

I trust my absence will not cause you any serious inconvenience.

Yours faithfully,

(Signature)

*　　*　　*

亲爱的 ××× 先生:

请原谅约翰今天不能到校。他昨天傍晚患了感冒,一直到夜里很迟才入睡。我觉得叫他去学校会影响其他孩子,现代请病假一天。如果明天他感觉好些，再让他到校。

您真诚的 ×××

2016 年 12 月 21 日

December 21, 2016

Dear Sir,

    Please excuse John's absence from school today. He had the snuffles yesterday evening and could not fall asleep until well into the night. I felt it would not have been fair to the other children to allow him to attend school. So I am writing to ask you for one day's sick leave and will let him resume his study if he feels better tomorrow.

Very truly yours,

×××

2. 请事假便条（Asking for business leave）

胡主任：

    我刚刚收到了一封我的母亲病重、催我立即回家的电报。我想从十月八日起请假 3 天，请求批准。

张小亮

2017 年 10 月 7 日

附：拍来电报一份

Oct. 7, 2017

Director Hu,

    A telegram has just come to hand saying that my mother is seriously ill and urging me to go home at once. Because of this I should very much like to have a leave of three days beginning on

Oct. 8. I hope that my request will be given due consideration.

Zhang Xiao-liang

Encl.: a telegram from my home

3. 续假便条（Asking for an extension of leave）

王老师：

我患重感冒未好，仍卧床不起。医生认为，还要休息 3 天才能到校学习。现附上所开的证明，请准予续假为盼。

学生：李勇

2017 年 7 月 5 日

附：医生证明

July 5, 2017

Teacher Wang,

I am still lying in bed with the bad cold and unable to get up. I enclose a certificate from the doctor who is attending on me, as he fear it will be another three days before I shall be able to resume my study. Please give an extension of leave for as many days.

Yours student,

Li Yong

Encl.: Doctor's Certificate of Advice

4. 请医生便条（Asking a doctor to come）

×××医生：

见条请即来外宾招待所 202 房间。大卫·贝克尔患重病需您帮忙。他急需立即治疗，务请速来。多谢。

×××

2017 年 10 月 19 日

Oct. 19, 2017

Dr. …,

Upon receipt of this note, please go to Room 202, Foreign Guest House, where David Becker is seriously ill and in urgent need of your service. Immediate treatment is absolutely necessary.

Be quick, and many thanks.

(Signature)

5. 取消会议便条（Cancelling a meeting）

×××博士：

因有一位从旧金山来的学者访问我校，原定明天召开的行政会议不得不取消。特此通知，并请转告各系主任。

×××

Dr. …,

Just a line to tell you that tomorrow's administrative meeting has to be cancelled because of a visit by a scholar from San Francisco. Please notify the Directors of other departments.

Yours,

(Signature)

6. 与同事约会便条（Making an appointment with a colleague）

亲爱的 ××× 先生：

请告诉我本周什么时候集体讨论今年的教学和科研工作为

宜？本次会议由您主持，谨此提醒。

×××

Dear Mr. ...,

　　Will you please tell me what time will be convenient for us to get together this week to discuss the teaching and research work for this year? I remind you that you will be in charge of the meeting.

Yours,

(Signature)

7. 转告电话便条（Transmitting a telephone message）

×××先生：

　　师范学院副院长王先生刚来电话，说今晚找您商谈艾伯拉姆斯博士访华的日程安排。请您在办公室等他。如不能见，请回电。

×××

Dear Mr. ...,

　　Mr. Wang, vice President of ... Normal College has just rung up, saying that he will come to see you this evening to talk about arranging our schedule for Dr. Abrams' visit to China. Please wait for him in your office, or ring him back if you can not meet with him.

(Signature)

8. 邀友来访便条（Asking a friend to call）

亲爱的×××：

　　如你最近有空儿见我，我十分感激。我有急事同你商量。

请给我打个电话或尽快来见我。

×××

Dear …,

I shall appreciate it if you can find time to see me in the very near future. I have something urgent to discuss with you. Please call, or come to see me as quickly as you can.

(Signature)

9. 请求介绍便条（Requesting an introduction）

亲爱的 ××× 书记：

我因公于明天乘机去上海，请为我给上海医科大学写封介绍信，以便我能得到一些帮助。

您的

×××

Dear Secretary …,

I am going to Shanghai on business by plane tomorrow. Will you please give me a letter of introduction to Shanghai Medical University, from which I expect to get some help in my business?

Yours ever,

(Signature)

10. 因迟复来信道歉便条（Apology for writing late）

亲爱的 ×××：

我想你一定会认为我不答复你五月十六日的来信是不可原

谅的疏忽,不过,我告诉你实情后,相信你一定会谅解的。你的信到来时,我正巧在杭州。你的信一直放在写字台上,直到我回来才看到。所以我现在要急着做的第一件事就是写这几行字来表达深深的歉意。

这次出去旅行饱览了许多美丽景色,下次见到你时将告诉你一切。

您的
× × ×

Dear …,

I am afraid that you will think me unpardonably negligent for not having answered your letter dated 16th May, but when I have told you the reason, I trust you will believe that the neglect was excusable. Your letter arrived while I was in Hangzhou, and it lay, therefore, on my desk until the moment I returned. Now the first thing I hasten to do is to write to you these few lines to express my deep regret.

I enjoyed many pleasant sights during my trip. I shall be pleased to give you an account when I see you next.

Yours,
(Signature)
…

11. 因故未能赴宴道歉便条（Apology for not coming to dinner）

亲爱的 × × × 先生：

因小女突然生病,昨晚未能应约赴宴,殊感歉疚,敬希原谅。

盼早晤面。

您的

× × ×

Dear Mr. ...,

Much to my regret I was unable to keep my promise to attend your dinner party yesterday, owing to the fact that my little daughter was suddenly taken ill.

Hoping to see you soon.

Yours truly,

(Signature)

...

12. 通知会议延期便条（Informing the meeting put off）

扬：

明天的会议因举办讲座延期召开，特告，并请转告有关人员。

大海

星期五下午

Friday afternoon

Dear Yang,

Just a line to tell you that tomorrow's meeting has been put off because of the lecture. Please notify others concerned.

Da-hai

* * *

大海：

感谢你的留言，会议准备在下星期一下午召开，是否合适？

扬明

星期五晚上

Friday evening

Dear Da-hai,

Thanks for your note. How about have the meeting next Monday afternoon?

Yang Ming

13. 代接电话留言（Message to one who is wanted to the phone）

史密斯先生：

布朗先生刚才打电话说，他很抱歉今晚不能来了。明天在展览会上见您。

张

1月7日下午5点15分

Dear Mr. Smith,

Mr. Brown just rang up to say that he very much regret he won't be able to come over this evening. He'll see you at the exhibition tomorrow.

Zhang

5:15 p.m. Jan. 7

14. 黑板留言（**Notes on the visitor's board**）

罗伯特：

　　我昨晚乘 14 次列车到达这里，现住在北京饭店三楼 4 号房间。有空请来叙谈。

吉姆

上午 9 点 30 分

9:30 a.m.

Robert,

　　I arrived last night by the Train No. 14. I am staying at Beijing Hotel (Room 304). Please come over and have a chat.

Jim

第二节　　通知（**Notice**）

　　通知是上级对下级、组织对成员布置工作、召开会议或传达事情时使用的一种应用文。平行单位之间有什么事情要互相协商、讨论，也可以互发通知。通知有两种，一种是书信式，寄出或发送，通知有关人员；另一种是布告形式，张贴通知。究竟采用哪种形式，应视实际需要。一般来说，对象为少量的分散人员，宜用书信的方式，其写法与普通书信的要求相同；如通知的对象为集中的较大范围以内的人员，例如学生、教师、会员以及读者、观众等，则宜采用布告的形式。我们这里所讲的属后一种。

　　这种通知一般在上方居中处写上 "Notice" 或 "NOTICE" 一词作为标志。正文的下面靠右下角写出通知的单位或人名，但也可放在正文上面。有时出通知的单位名称用在本文的开头，这样就不需要另外注明。出通知的单位以及被通知的对象一般都用第三人称。如果正文前用了称呼用语，则用第二人称表示通知对象。

1. 会议通知（Meeting notice）

通　　知

兹定于四月六日星期一下午三点在校会议室召开校学术委员会全体会员会议，讨论校际学术交流问题，请准时出席。

校学术委员会

2017 年 4 月 4 日

The University Commission of Academic Research
NOTICE

All the members of the University Commission of Academic Research are requested to meet in the University conference room on Monday, April 6 at 3:00 p.m. to discuss questions of inter–collegiate academic exchanges.

April 4, 2017

2. 报告会延期通知（Notice to put off a report meeting）

通　　知

接外事办公室通知，托马斯·杰弗逊大学副校长、杰弗逊医学院院长约瑟夫·冈纳拉博士不能按期到中国访问。他的关于医学院教育的报告将推迟到 2017 年 4 月 22 日（下星期四）下午 2 时在学校礼堂举行。

特此通知。

教务处

2017 年 4 月 10 日

NOTICE

The Foreign Affairs Office has informed us that Dr. Joseph Gonnella, Dean & Vice President of Thomas Jefferson Medical College, Thomas Jefferson University will be unable to travel to China as planned. His report on medical education has been rescheduled for next Thursday, April 22, 2017 at 2:00 p.m. in the school auditorium.

Teaching Affairs Department

April 10, 2017

3. 选举结果公告（Proclamation of election results）

公　　告

×××教授于 2017 年 10 月 12 日当选为××医科大学公共卫生系主任，现予公告。

××医科大学

校长办公室

2017 年 10 月 15 日

PROCLAMATION

It is hereby proclaimed that on October 12, 2017 Prof. ... was elected to Dean of the Public Health Faculty, ... Medical University.

The President's Office

... Medical University

October 15, 2017

4. 免职通知（Notice of dismissal）

免 职 通 知

经董事会投票一致通过,免去 ××× 先生院长办公室主任职务,现予公布。

董事会办公室

2017 年 5 月 20 日

NOTICE OF DISMISSAL

It is hereby proclaimed that the Board of Directors has unanimously voted to dismiss Mr. ... from the post of Director of the President's Office.

The Director's Office

May 20, 2017

5. 任职通知（Notice of an appointment）

任 职 通 知

现任命 ××× 为外事办公室主任,特予公布。

×× 医学院院长

×××

2017 年 10 月 6 日

NOTICE OF APPOINTMENT

It is hereby declared that the President of … Medical College has appointed Mr. … Director of Foreign Affairs Office.

…, M.D.

President

… Medical College

October 6, 2017

6. 授予荣誉职称的通知(Notice of honorary appointment)

授予荣誉职称的通知

中国 × × 医学院授予美国费城托马斯·杰弗逊大学相关卫生学院院长劳伦斯·艾伯拉姆斯博士名誉教授称号,特予通知。

× × 医学院院长

× × ×

2017 年 7 月 3 日

NOTICE OF HONORARY APPOINTMENT

… Medical College of the People's Republic of China confers a honorary professorship on Dr. Lawrence Abrams, Dean of College of Allied Health Sciences, Thomas Jefferson University, Philadelphia, the United States of America.

..., M.D.

President

... Medical College

3rd, July 2017

7. 聘任通知(Notice of appointment)

聘 任 通 知

兹聘请多伦多大学临床生化系研究生教育教授 ××× 博士为 ×× 医学院客座教授,特予通知。

×× 医学院院长

×××

2017 年 8 月 23 日

NOTICE OF APPOINTMENT

Dr. ..., Professor of Graduate Studies in the Department of Clinical Biochemistry, University of Toronto, is appointed to a visiting professorship at ... Medical College.

..., M.D.

President

... Medical College

August 23rd, 2017

8. 放假通知（Notice giving a holiday）

放 假 通 知

　　明天国庆节，学校将放假7天。全体教职工和学生可参加我校举行的各种庆祝活动。十月八日照常上课。特此通知。

院长办公室

2017 年 9 月 30 日

NOTICE

　　Tomorrow being National Day, there will be no school. All teachers, staff members and students are expected to take part in the celebrations held in our school. Classed will resume on October 8th as the usual hour.

President's Office

September 30, 2017

9. 出生通知（Notice of birth）

通 知

　　×××先生和夫人高兴地宣布他们的儿子在 2017 年 4 月 27 日出生。

NOTICE

　　Mr. & Mrs. ... have the pleasure of announcing the birth of their son on the twenty–seventh of April 2017.

10. 讣告（死亡通知）（Obituary notice）

讣　告

×××夫人及其子女最沉痛地宣布她尊敬的丈夫和她们敬爱的父亲于2017年12月25日逝世。遗体告别仪式定于2017年12月30日下午4时30分在芬德殡仪馆举行。

NOTICE

Mrs. … and her children announce with the deepest sorrow the parting of Prof. … their respected and beloved husband and father on the 25th of December, 2017. The farewell service will be held at 4:30 p.m. Saturday, 30th of December, 2017 at Fende Funeral Parlour.

11. 住址变动通知（Notice of a new address）

通　知

×××先生和夫人宣布从2017年5月4日起变更新地址如下：

承德市双桥区翠桥路123号

邮政编码：067000

电话：332691

NOTICE

Mr. and Mrs. … wish to announce their new address as follows: from 4th May, 2017.

123 Cuiqiao Road

Shuangqiao District

Chengde 067000
Phone: 332691

12. 参观的通知（Notice of a visit）

通　　知

　　定于 7 月 18 日（星期六）组织到遵化市清东陵参观。凡愿意前往参观者，请早晨 5 时 45 分在办公楼前运动场集合，6 时乘车前往。

学生会
2017 年 7 月 12 日

NOTICE

　　ATTENTION. A visit to the East Qing Dynasty Tombs in Zun Hua County is being arranged for Saturday, July 18. Those who wish to go, please be on the sports grounds in front of the Office Building by 5:45 a.m. The bus will leave promptly at 6:00 a.m.

Student Association
July 12, 2017

证明书和公证书（Certificate）

第一节　证明书（Certificate）

证明书涉及面广，凡是证明一个人的身份、经历或某件事情真相的文件，都是证明书，如出生证明书，死亡证明书以及学历证明书等。英文证明书的书写格式较普通书信来说要简单得多，它不需用收信人姓名、地址和结束语，通常在纸笺的上方先注明 Certificate（证明书）字样，然后直接将要证明的内容写上，最后署上自己的名字或单位名称。但有关，某人的缺点一般不写在证明信上，而只是附一句"如欲知详情，请另函询问，证明人乐于奉告"。

1. 身份证明（Identity Certificate）

证　明　书

兹证明玛丽·D·哈瑞森，女，21 岁，美国密执安州人，确系我校留学生。

×××大学

2017 年 5 月 25 日

Certificate

This is to certify that Mary D. Harrison, female, aged 21, from Michigan, the United States of America, is undoubtedly a foreign student of our university.

… University
May 25, 2017

*　　　*　　　*

身份证明书

兹证明×××博士，美国籍，男，43岁，系我院聘请的心脏病学专家，他持有美国护照，现住我院外宾招待所545房间，×××博士已向××市公安局外事处申报了临时户口。

××医学院外事办公室主任

×××

2017年11月16日

IDENTITY CERTIFICATE

This is to certify that Dr. …, an American citizen, male, age 43, is a cardiologist in the employment of our college. He holds an American passport and lives in the Foreign Guest House of our College, Room No.545. Dr. … has a registered temporary residence with the Foreign Affairs Department of … Security Bureau.

(Signature)

Director
Foreign Affairs Office
... Medical College
November 16, 2017

2. 毕业证书（Graduation certificate）

<h1 style="text-align:center">毕 业 证 书</h1>

×××（男）系北京市人，现年22岁，于2017年8月在××医学院毕业，学制五年，按德、智、体全面发展的要求，考察合格，准予毕业。

×× 医学院院长
×××（签字）
2017 年 8 月 8 日

GRADUATION CERTIFICATE

..., male, born in Beijing, 22 years old, graduated from ... Medical College in August, 2017, after five years study. He has satisfied all moral, intellectual and physical requirements. Graduation is approved.

(Signature)
..., M.D.
President
... Medical College
August 8, 2017

*　　*　　*

毕 业 证 书

第 82008 号

学生 × × × ，性别女，天津市人，1992 年 3 月 22 日生，2012 年 9 月 1 日至 2017 年 7 月 31 日在本校医学系五年制本科学习期满，完成学校教学计划的全部课程，考试成绩及格，准予毕业。

× × × 医学院院长

× × × （签字）

2017 年 10 月 4 日

DIPLOMA

…, female, born on March 22, 1992, native of Tianjin, was an undergraduate student majoring in medicine in the Department of Medicine, … Medical College from September 1, 2012 to July 31, 2017. She has completed all the prescribed five year undergraduate courses, passed all the examinations and is entitled to graduate from … Medical College.

(Signature)

…

No.820018

President

… Medical College

Issued on: October 4, 2017

3. 研究生毕业证书（Graduation certificate for the master degree）

毕 业 证 书

×××（男），系北京市人，在我院神经外科学专业学习二年半，修业期满，完成硕士学位的全部课程，考试合格，准予毕业。

×××医学院院长

×××（签字）

2017 年 10 月 4 日

GRADUATION CERTIFICATE

..., male, born in Beijing, after two and a half years study in neurosurgery at ... Medical College and completion of a graduate training program, has passed all courses and examinations for the Master's Degree.

(Signature)

..., M.D.

President

... Medical College

October 4, 2017

4. 研究生学位证书（Certificate of master degree）

研究生学位证书

×××（男），系北京市人，1987 年 8 月 18 日生，在我院已通过硕士学位的课程考试，成绩合格，根据《中华人民共和国学位条例》的规定，授予医学硕士学位。

> ××医学院院长
> ×××（签字）
> 2017 年 11 月 18 日

CERTIFICATE OF MASTER DEGREE

..., male, born in Beijing on August 18,1987, has passed the courses and examinations for the Master's degree in ... Medical College. In accordance with academic rules of the People's Republic of China, the Master's Degree of Medicine is hereby awarded.

> (Signature)
> ..., M.D.
> President
> ... Medical College
> November 18, 2017

5. 奖状（Certificate of merit）

奖 状

医学系学生×××，学习勤奋，工作认真，为人正直，品德高尚，忠于职守，各科成绩一贯优秀，连续三年被评为模范学生，特发此状，以资表彰。

> ××医学院（印）
> 2017 年 8 月 4 日

CERTIFICATE OF MERIT

..., a student of Medical Department, has distinguished herself by diligent, accurate, moral and conscientious discharge of all her duties. She has received high marks on all subjects in the examination. She has been cited as a model student for three years in succession. This certificate of merit is hereby given in commendation of her.

... Medical college

August 4, 2017

6. 介绍信(Introduction Letter)

介　绍　信

兹证明×××先生,1992年2月3日生,是××医学院全日制八年级学生。他非常愿意到贵院(医院)攻读博士学位。如能安排,不胜感激。

真诚的

×××

2017年3月7日

Introduction Letter

This is to confirm Mr. ... born on Feburary 3, 1992, is enrolled as a full-time student of medicine at ... Medical College. He is in his 8th-year term and would very much like to come to your medical school (hospital) to pursue his Ph.D.degree.

I would appreciate it if you could arrange this for Mr. …

Sincerely,

(Signature)

…

March 7, 2017

7. 医生证明书（Doctor's certificate）

医生证明书

兹证明病人 ×××，男，40 岁，因患急性阑尾炎于 2017 年 3 月 10 日住院。经急症手术和 10 天治疗现已痊愈。将于 2017 年 3 月 20 日出院，建议在家休息一周后再上班。

医生：× × ×

2017 年 3 月 19 日

Doctor's certificate

March 19, 2017

This is to certify that the patient, …, male, age 40, was admitted to our hospital on March 10, 2017, suffering from acute appendicitis. After emergency operation and ten days of treatment, he has completely recovered and will be discharged on March 20, 2017. It is suggested that he rests for one week at home before resuming his work.

(Signature)

…, M.D.

8. 诊断证明（Medical certificate）

诊 断 证 明

　　兹证明病人×××，男，41岁，因患急性阑尾炎，于2017年12月11日住院。经立即施行手术和10天治疗，现已痊愈。将于2017年12月21日出院。建议在家休息一个星期后再上班工作。

医生：×××

2017 年 12 月 20 日

Medical certificate

Dec. 20, 2017

　　This is to certify that the patient, ..., male, aged 41, was admitted to our hospital on Dec. 11, 2001 for suffering from acute appendicitis. After immediate operation and ten days of treatment, he has got complete recovery and will be discharged on Dec. 21, 2017. It is suggested that he rests for one week at home before resuming his work.

Dr. ...

9. 病假证明（Certificate for sick leave）

病 假 证 明

　　×××先生，26岁，高热39℃，喉痛严重。建议休息3天，必要时再来医院复查。

特此证明。

主治医生：××

2017 年 2 月 12 日

Certificate for sick leave

March 12, 2017

This is to certify that Mr. ... aged 26, has a high fever of 39℃ and a very bad sore throat. We advise that he takes a three–day rest and if necessary, comes back for a check by that time.

Physician in Charge

(Signature)

10. 入院证明（Certificate for admission）

入 院 证 明

兹证明 ××× 先生正患肺炎，应住院进行进一步检查和治疗。

医生：×××

2017 年 6 月 5 日

Certificate for admission

June 5, 2017

This is to certify that Mr. ... is suffering from pneumonia and should be admitted to our hospital for further examination and treatment.

Dr. ...

11. 体格检查证明（Certificate of physical examination）

体格检查证明书

兹证明×××,男性,25岁,经检查无任何传染性疾病,身体健康,每天可以胜任8小时工作。

医生：×××

2017 年 3 月 6 日

Certificate of physical examination

This is to certify that Mr. …, male, age 25, examined by me, is free of all infectious diseases. He is in good health and capable of working eight hours day.

(Signature)

…, M.D.

March 6, 2017

第二节   公证书（Notarized certificate）

公证书是指被授予权利的公证机关对某人或某事的实际情况所做的书面证明,它的书写形式要比一般证明书严格。通常的写法是先将年限代号、公证机关代号和公证书编号依次并排写在右上角,然后另起一行,直接写明要证明的内容。最后在正文末尾下一行的右边,分别署上公证机关的全称、公证人姓名和发文日期。

书写公证书要严肃认真,引用材料必须真实、可靠,有凭有据,而且语言还应简洁、清楚。

1. 出生证明（**Birth Certificate**）

出生证明书

（01）宁公证字第 1232 号

吴光祖，男，一九五八年五月二十一日在江苏南京市出生。父吴义德，母史美琴，特此证明。

中华人民共和国江苏省南京市公证处

公证员　肖南

二〇一七年九月二十日

Birth Certificate

(01) Ning Zi, No. 1232

This is to certify that Guang–zhu Wu, male, was born on May 21, 1958, in Nanjing City, Jiangsu Province. Guang–zhu's father is Yi–de Wu, and Guang–zhu's mother is Mei–qin Shi.

Nanjing Notary Public Office

Jiangsu Province

The People's Republic of China

Notary：Xiao Nan

September 20, 2017

2. 死亡证明（**Death certificate**）

死亡证明书

（01）宁公证字第 859 号

兹证明吴义德，男，一九五四年七月生于江苏南京，于二〇一六年十一月二十七日病故。

中华人民共和国南京市公证处

公证员　肖南

二〇一七年二月十九日

Death certificate

(01) Ning Zi, No. 859

This is to certify that Yi–de Wu died of illness on November 27, 2016.Yi–de Wu, male, native of Nanjing, Jiangsu Province, was born in July, 1954.

Nanjing Notary Public Office

The People's Republic of China

Notary: Xiao Nan

Feburary 19, 2017

3. 结婚证书（Marriage certificate）

结　婚　证　书

兹证明×××（男，1955 年 3 月 24 日出生）和×××（女，1956 年 7 月 18 日出生）于 1983 年 9 月 5 日在中国××市结婚。

中华人民共和国

××市公证处

公证员 ×××

2017 年 11 月 9 日

Marriage certificate

This is to certify that … (male, born on March 24, 1955) and … (female, born on July 18, 1956) were married on September 5, 1983 in …, China.

… Notary Public Office

The People's Republic of China

(sealed)

Notary: (Signature)

(sealed)

Dated this 9th day of November, 2017

4. 学历证明（Schooling record certificate）

学历证明书

兹证明×××先生，男，××市人，生于1985年4月，系生理学教研室讲师。2007年毕业于××医学院，获理学学士学位；2010年毕业于北京医学院，获理学硕士学位；2014年获美国宾夕法尼亚大学哲学博士学位，2016年获国家科技奖。

中华人民共和国

××市公证处

公证员×××

2017年8月10日

Schooling certificate

This is to certify that Mr. ..., male, born in ... City, in April 1985, is a lecturer in the physiology Department. He graduated from ... Medical College in 2007 with a Bachelor of Science degree and completed his postgraduate course in Beijing Medical College in July 2010 for the degree of Master of Science. He received his Doctor of philosophy degree from University of Pennsylvania in the United States of America in 2014. He received a state science and technology award in 2016.

(Signature)
Public Notary,
... Notary Public Office.
The people's Republic of China
Dated this 10 day of August, 2017

医务文件（Medical document）

第一节 入院记录（Admission notes）

1. 急性阑尾炎（Acute appendicitis）

入院治疗证

现证明密尔顿先生，男，43岁，患急性阑尾炎，建议立即住院施行手术。

外科主治医师陈叶德

（医院公章）

2017年10月23日

Admission Certificate

Oct. 23, 2017

This is to certify that Mr. Milton, male, aged 43, is suffering from acute appendicitis. It is suggested that he should be immediately hospitalized and operated on.

Chen Ye-de

Surgeon in Charge

(Seal)

2. 慢性肾盂肾炎急性发作（Chronic pyelonephritis with acute attacks）

入 院 记 录

患者，女，42 岁，未婚。因尿急尿频和右侧腰痛 20 余天，于 2017 年 8 月 26 日入院。

20 多天前，她开始尿急、尿频，几乎每小时小便一次，伴轻度右侧腰痛，故 2017 年 8 月 10 日到某医院验小便。

显微镜检：每高倍视野白细胞 6~8 个，脓细胞 8~12 个。

尿培养：分离出变形杆菌，对氯霉素敏感。

药物治疗 7 天后，尿频显著减少，但仍感体弱，故来罗蒂芬克医院进一步治疗。

病期无发热、咳嗽及呕吐。大便正常。

2015 年及 2016 年 8 月两次类似症状发作，诊断为肾盂肾炎。

月经周期正常。

体格检查：体温 37℃，脉搏 82 次 /min，呼吸 20 次 /min，血压 120/70mmHg（16/9kPa）。

一般情况好，皮肤无黄染。无浅淋巴结肿大。心脏的边界未扩大，无杂音，肺阴性。腹部柔软，肝、脾未扪及，右肾区有压痛。肠鸣音正常。脊柱及四肢无异常。膝反射存在。无病理反射。

血常规化验如下：血红蛋白 125g/L，白细胞 5 300/mm^3，中性 63%，淋巴 35%，单核 2%。

小便化验：每高倍视野白细胞 4~6 个，脓细胞 6~8 个。

诊断：慢性肾盂肾炎急性发作

签字: × × ×

日期: 2017 年 8 月 26 日

Admission Notes

A 42-year-old unmarried female gained admission to the hospital on August 26, 2017, because of urgency and frequency of micturition and a right lumbago, which have each lasted for over twenty days.

More than twenty days ago, she began experiencing urgency and frequency of micturition, urinating almost once an hour with a slight right lumbago at the same time; she, therefore, went to a hospital for a urine test on August 10, 2017.

Microscopy: WBC 6~8/HPF. Pus cell 8~12/HPF.

Findings of urine culture: Bacilli proteus, which are sensitive to chloromycetin, were isolated.

After a 7-day course of treatment with the medicine, there was a considerable decrease in the frequency of urination. As she still felt weak, she came to Rotifunk Hospital for further treatment.

She has not suffered from fever, cough or vomiting and there has been nothing specific in her stools in the course of her illness either.

In the two similar attacks, which happened in 2015 and in August 2016 respectively, the diagnosis of pyelonephritis was established.

Her menstrual cycle is normal.

PE T: 37℃; P: 82/min; R: 20/min; BP: 120/70mmHg (16/9kPa).

General condition is good, and no jaundice on skin. Superficial lymph nodes not felt. Heart not enlarged. No murmur heard. Lungs negative. Abdomen soft. Liver and spleen impalpable. Tenderness over right kidney region detectable. Bowel sounds normal. Spine and extremities not abnormal. Knee jerk present. No pathological reflex observable.

Findings of routine blood test: Hb 125g/L, WBC 5 300/mm^3, N 63%, L 35%, M 2%.

Findings of urine test: WBC 4~6/HPF. Pus cells 6~8/HPF.

Diagnosis:　Chronic Pyelonephritis with Acute Attacks

Signature: Dr. … (M.D.)

Date: August 26, 2017

3. 心脏病（Heart attack）

入 院 记 录

患者,女,30 岁,已婚。劳累后心悸 20 年左右,因畏寒、发热、呼吸困难和踝水肿半个月,于 2017 年 4 月 15 日收入罗蒂芬克医院。

约 20 年前,患者激烈活动后第一次感到心悸,而后上述症状逐渐加剧。10 年前上楼梯或工作时气喘,被迫求医。并发现心脏杂音,诊断为心脏病,未予治疗。直到半个月前,她仍能从事轻微劳动,那时患重感冒,畏寒、咳嗽无痰、发热、全身痛。近日来,因上腹膨胀、恶心、呕吐和踝水肿而病情加重,故不能平卧。同时心悸、呼吸困难进一步加剧,故来院就医。

患病期间食欲差,小便减少,大便正常,未服地高克辛类药物,无阵发性夜间哮喘。

自童年起,常患喉痛,关节痛。

15 岁初潮,正常。19 岁结婚,1 年后正常分娩 1 男孩,现身体好,10 岁。

无心脏病及与此有关的家庭病史。

体检:体温 38℃,脉搏 108 次 /min,呼吸 24 次 /min,血压 120/80mmHg（16/11kPa）。

发育正常,中度营养,神志清醒,半坐位,呈急性病容,呼吸困难,轻度发绀,两颊潮红。浅淋巴结无肿大。皮肤及巩膜无黄染。咽稍充血。颈软,活动自如。气管居中,无甲状腺肿大,但颈静脉充盈。胸部对称,肺清晰。心尖搏动于第五肋间,在左锁骨中线上。心搏100~108次/min,期外收缩7~8次/min,心尖区可闻及递增性的舒张期隆隆性杂音,较局限,不传导。主动脉瓣区第二心音等于肺动脉瓣区第二心音。腹部平软,肝于肋下5cm处可触及,质软,无压痛,肝颈回流阳性。脾未触及,腹部未触及肿块,无移动性浊音。肾区无压痛。肠鸣音正常。脊柱、四肢无异常,下肢指压性水肿明显,膝反射存在。无病理性反射。肛门及外阴未检查。

X线、心电图和化验结果如下:

(1) 红细胞沉降率: 15mm/h

(2) 抗链"O": 200单位

(3) 胸片报告: 左心房、右心室扩大,肺动脉突出。食管向后移位,符合二尖瓣心脏病的诊断。

(4) 心电图显示:

① 心室期外收缩

② P波宽大于0.12mm, $RV_1+SV_5=1.5mv$

诊断: 风湿性心脏病

二尖瓣狭窄

右心室扩大

心力衰竭

室性早搏

签名:×××

日期:2017年4月15日

Admission Notes

The patient, a 30-year-old married female, was admitted to Rotifunk Hospital on April 15, 2017, complaining of palpitations, which had been caused by hard work and had lasted some twenty years, and of chills, fever, dyspnea and edema of the ankle, which had all been continuing for half a month.

About twenty years ago, the patient suffered for the first time from palpitations, which occurred after vigorous physical exercise, and which have been gradually worsening ever since. Ten years ago, she began to experience dyspnea while going upstairs or doing work; therefore, she had accepted medical treatment. A cardiac murmur was subsequently discovered and a diagnosis of heart disease was given, which was not treated. Nevertheless, she had been capable of doing light work until half a month ago, when she caught a bad cold, which was accompanied by chills, cough non-productive of sputum. In the last few days, her condition has become aggravated by epigastric distention, nausea, vomiting and edema of the ankles and she was thus unable to lie supine. Palpitations and dyspnea were further aggravated at the same time. For this reason, she had to come to the hospital for treatment.

In the course of her illness, she has had anorexia and oliguria without abnormal bowel motions; she has not taken digoxin or its equivalent; and she has not suffered from paroxysmal nocturnal asthma.

She has often had laryngalgia and arthralgia since her childhood.

Her menarche began when she was fifteen and it was regular. She got married at the age of nineteen. A year later, she normally delivered a baby boy, who is now ten years old and healthy.

There is no cardiac disease or other related disorders in her family medical history.

PE T: 38℃ ; P: 108/min; R: 24/min; BP: 120/80mmHg (16/11kPa).

Normally developed. Moderately nourished. Mind clear. In a semi sitting position. Acutely ill-looking, showing dyspnea, slight cyanosis and flushing. Superficial lymph nodes not palpable. No jaundice on skin or sclerae. Pharynx slightly congested. Neck soft and supple. Trachea in midline. No thyroid enlargement, but with engorgement of jugular veins. Chest not asymmetrical. Lungs clear. Apex beat felt in 5th inter-costal space along left midclavicular line. Heart beat fluctuated between 100/min. and 108/min., extrasystoles occurring 7~8/min. A rumbling, crescendo diastolic murmur heard over apex, rather localized, not transmitted elsewhere. A2 equal to P2. Abdomen flat and soft. Liver palpable 5cm below costal margin with soft consistency and free from tenderness. Hepatojugular reflux positive. Spleen not felt. Abdomen free of any mass or mobile dullness. No tendrness in kidney. Bowel sounds not abnormal. No deformity of spine or extremities. Marked pitting edema in lower extremities. Knee jerks present. No pathological reflex. Anus and external genitalia not examined.

Findings of X-rays, ECG and laboratory test presented below:

(1) ESR 15mm/h

(2) ASO 200U

(3) Chest fluoroscopy: Left atrium and right ventricle enlarged, with prominent pulmonary artery, and esophagus displaced posteriorly, compatible with diagnosis of mitral valve heart disease.

(4) ECG shows: a. ventricular premature beat

b. width of p>0.12mm. $RV_1+SV_5=1.5mv$

Diagnosis: Rheumatic Heart Disease

Mitral Stenosis

Right Ventricular Enlargement

Heart Failure

Ventricular Premature Beat

Signature: Dr. …, (M.D.)

Date: April 15, 2017

4. 慢性十二指肠溃疡（Chronic duodenal ulcer）

入 院 记 录

患者，女性，成年，未婚，因间歇性腹痛 6 年，近 3 天加剧，于 2017 年 2 月 14 日入院。

6 年前，她开始患上腹痛，以后每年发作 1 次，持续数天至数周不等，常与饮食不慎有关。有时夜间腹痛，偶尔痛醒；食物与碱性药物均可缓解疼痛。

近年来，间歇缩短，发作更频繁。3 天前上腹痛发作，伴频繁呕吐食物，无血。

病程中无发热、黄染，有体弱、纳差。大、小便正常。

以往月经史和生育史不详。

体检：体温 37℃，脉搏 90 次/min，呼吸 20 次/min，血压 120/80mmHg（16~11kPa）。

发育正常，神志清醒，呈急性病容。皮肤和巩膜无黄染。浅淋巴结无肿大。咽喉正常，颈软、活动自如，气管居中，甲状腺不肿大。胸廓对称，心界未及扩大，无杂音，肺呼吸音清。腹平软，上腹有压痛，无肿块。肝于肋缘下 1cm 处可触及，脾不可触及。肠鸣音正常。膝反射减退。无病理反射。

X 线检查及化验结果如下：

（1）钡餐：十二指肠冠部变形，表示溃疡存在。

（2）血常规：血红蛋白 118g/L，白细胞 6 800/mm^3，中性粒细胞 62%，淋巴细胞 36%，单核细胞 2%。

诊断：慢性十二指肠溃疡

签名：×××

日期：2017 年 2 月 14 日

Admission Notes

The patient, an unmarried adult female, was admitted to the hospital on February 14, 2017, complaining of a 6-year intermittent abdominalgia which has been worsening in the last three days.

Six years ago, she developed an epigastralgia which has occurred once a year since that time, persisting for days or even for weeks at each time and has often been associated with dietary indiscretion. Sometimes she has nocturnal abdominalgia, which is at times severe enough to wake up the patient from sleep, but both food and alkaline medicines relieve her of the pain.

In recent years, the intervals between attacks have become shorter and the attacks more frequent. Three days ago, there was a relapse of the epigastralgia accompanied by frequent vomiting of gastric contents, but not by blood.

In the course of her illness there has been no fever or jaundice, but weakness and anorexia. Bowel motions and micturiton are normal.

Past menstrual and obstetric history is unknown.

PE T: 37℃ ; P: 90/min ; R: 20/min; BP: 120/80mmHg (16~11kPa).

Normally developed. Mentally clear, but acutely ill-looking. No jaundice on skin or sclerae. Superficial lymph nodes not palpable. Pharynx and larynx not abnormal. Neck soft and supple. Trachea in midline. Thyroid not enlarged. Chest symmetrical. Heart not enlarged, without murmur. Lungs clear. Abdomen soft and flat with tenderness in epigastrium but with no mass. Liver not impalpable 1cm below costal margin. Spleen not felt. Bowel sounds not abnormal. Knee jerks less active. No pathological reflexes found.

X-ray and laboratory findings reveal:

(1) Barium meal: Duodenal cap deformed confirming and /or showing the presence of duodenal ulcer.

(2) Blood picture: Hb 118g/L, WBC 6 800/mm^3, N 62%, L 36%, M 2%.

Diagnosis　Chronic Duodenal Ulcer

Signature　　　　Dr. ... (M.D.)

Date　　February 14, 2017

5. 泌尿道感染（Urinary tract infection）

入 院 记 录

患者，男，42 岁，外交官，因多饮、多尿、排尿疼痛约 15 天，于 2017 年 4 月 20 日入院。

15 天前，患者小便量多，伴尿急、尿痛，故前往弗里敦某医院验尿，发现尿糖阳性，有金黄色葡萄球菌。每天小便 8~9 次，每次约 200ml。进食比以往略多，有时仍感饥饿。患者不能说出这种情况有多久。通常饮水不多，但近来增多。近两年体重减轻 10kg。皮肤无瘙痒。

患病期间一般情况尚可，大便正常。

5 年前排尿困难，"诊断为膀胱炎"。

家族中无糖尿病及有关病史。

体检：体温 37 ℃，脉搏 82 次/min，呼吸 18 次/min，血压 120/80mmHg（16~11kPa）。

一般尚好，肥胖体型，皮肤无黄染及脓疱，无浅淋巴结肿大。头和耳鼻喉正常。颈软活动自如，气管居中，无甲状腺肿大。心脏边界未扩大，无杂音。肺阴性，腹软无压痛，肝、脾未扪及，肾区无压痛，肠鸣音正常。脊柱及四肢无畸形。膝反射正常。无病理反射。

X 线及化验检查结果如下：

尿：

尿分析：颜色：黄色；透明度：清晰；反应：酸性；蛋白：阴性；糖：（＋）

显微镜检查：白细胞 3~5/ 高倍视野

尿培养：分离出金黄色葡萄球菌

空腹血糖：8mmol/L

肝功能：血清胆红素：6mmol/L。麝香草酚浊度试验 4 个单位。硫酸锌浊度试验 8 个单位。谷丙转氨酶 60 个单位。

心电图：正常。

胸部 X 线透视检查：肺野清晰，心脏大小正常，膈肌平滑。

诊断：轻度糖尿病

泌尿道感染

签字：×××

日期：2017 年 4 月 20 日

Admission Notes

The patient, a 42-year-old male diplomat, was admitted on April 20, 2017 because of excessive water intake, polyuria and urodynia for about fifteen days.

The patient reported that fifteen days before he had much urine associated with frequency of mictrition and urodynia, for which he went to a hospital in Freetown for a urinary test. The urinalysis revealed positive glycosuria and staphylococci aureus. He urinated eight or nine times a day, passing about 200 ml. urine each time.

He ate slightly more than before, but sometimes he still felt hungry. He did not know the exact duration of the condition. Usually he felt that he did not drink much water, but his water intake had increased recently. He had lost 10kg. within the last two years. He did not feel itching of the skin.

His general condition remained fair and feces normal throughout his illness.

Five years ago, he had dysuria, which 'was diagnosed as cystitis.'

There was no family medical history of diabetes or relevant disorders.

PE T: 37℃ ; P: 82/min.; R: 18/min ; BP: 120/80mmHg (16~11kPa).

General condition fair. Obese somatotype. No apparent jaundice or pustules over skin. Superficial lymph nodes impalpable. Head and ENT not abnormal. Neck soft and supple. Trachea in midline. No enlargment of thyroid. Heart not enlarged, no murmur heard. Lung negative. Abdomen soft with no tenderness. Liver and spleen not felt. No tenderness in kidney area. Bowel sounds not abnormal. No deformity of spine or extremities. Knee jerk not abnormal, no pathological reflexes elicited.

Roentgenographic and laboratory findings shown below:

Urine:

Urinalysis: colour: straw; transparency: clear; reaction: acid; protein: negative; glucose: +;

Microscopy: WBC 3~5/HPF;

Culture: staphylococci aureus isolated.

FBS: 8 mmol/L

Liver function: SB: 6mmol/L; TTT: 4 units; ZnTT: 8 units; SGPT: 60 units.

ECG: normal.

Chest fluoroscopy: Lung fields clear, heart normal in size, diaphragm smooth.

Diagnosis: Mild Diabetes

Urinaty Tract Infection

Signature: Dr. … (M.D.)

Date: April 20, 2017

6. 大叶性肺炎（Lobar pneumonia）

入院记录

患者，女，28 岁，已婚。因发热、咳嗽 6 天，于 2017 年 5 月 3 日入院。

6 天前开始发热、咳嗽、吐黏液痰，至今未治疗。近 3 天，持续高烧，咳嗽加剧，吐铁锈色痰，胸痛，随呼吸加剧。

患病期，乏力，食欲差，大、小便正常。

既往体健，很少就医。

家中无人患结核病，患者是否有与结核病人密切交往史不详。

体检：体温 39℃，脉搏 107 次 /min，呼吸 26 次 /min，血压 110/70mmHg（15/9kPa）。

发育正常，营养不良。急性病容，神志清楚。无发绀，皮肤无疹子及紫癜，无浅淋巴结肿大。头颅正常，巩膜无黄染。颈活动自如，甲状腺未肿大。气管无偏移，颈静脉不充盈。胸廓对称，右上胸语颤略有增强，可听到许多中小湿性啰音。心跳正常，无杂音。腹平软，无触痛，肝、脾未触及，肠鸣音正常。脊柱和四肢无异常。双侧膝反射活跃。无病理反射。

血常规：红细胞 450 万 /mm^3，血红蛋白 145g/L，白细胞 21 000/mm^3，中性粒细胞 80%，淋巴细胞 19%，嗜酸细胞 1%。

血小板计数：15 万 /mm^3。

胸部 X 线透视：右上肺有大片状阴影。

诊断：大叶性肺炎

签字：×××

日期：2017 年 5 月 3 日

Admission Notes

A 28-year-old married female was admitted to the hospital on May 3, 2017, because of a 6-day fever and cough.

Six days ago, she began running a fever and having a bad cough productive of mucous sputum, for which she has not taken any medical treatment up to now. In the past three days, she has been having a persistent high fever, an exacerbated cough productive of rusty sputum and a thoracalgia intensified with respirations.

During her illness, she has been weak and has had a poor appetite without specific urine or stools.

She has been in good health and has seldom consulted physicians in the past.

There is no tuberculosis in her family medical history and she does not know of any intimate exposure to patients with this disease either.

PE T: 39℃; P: 107/min; R: 26/min.; BP: 110/70mmHg (15/9kPa).

Well developed, poorly nourished. Acutely ill-looking, still mentally clear. No cyanosis. No eruption or purpura over skin. Superficial lymph nodes not palpable. Skull and head organs not remarkable. No jaundice on sclera. Neck soft and supple. Thyroid not enlarged. Trachea not deviated. No engorgement of jugular veins.

Chest symmetrical. Tactile fremitus exaggerated slightly over the right upper chest and a lot of small and moderate moist rales heard here. Heart beat regular with no murmur. Abdomen flat, soft and free from tenderness. Liver and spleen impalpable. Intestinal peristaltic sounds normal. No abnormality detected in spine or limbs. Knee jerks of both sides active. no pathological reflexes elicited.

Routine blood test: RBC 4 500 000/mm^3; Hb 145g/L; WBC 21 000/mm^3; N 80%; L 19%; E 1%.

Platelet count: 150 000/mm^3.

Chest fluoroscopy: A big patchy density over upper right lung.

Diagnosis: Lobar Pneumonia

Signature: Dr. ... (M.D.)

Date: May 3, 2017

7. 冠状动脉性心脏病（Coronary heart disease）

入 院 记 录

患者，男性，60 岁，已婚。因心悸、胸痛 2 个月于 2017 年 5 月 13 日入院。

今年 3 月以来患者用力时常感心悸和胸痛，后者放射到左肩及左臂。每次发作持续约 5min。有窒息感，似重物压在胸口。轻咳，发作时咳少量黏液痰。因以前未治疗，上述症状本周加剧，又腿肿，所以来此治疗。

患病期间乏力，食欲好，大、小便正常。

既往体健，未患过风湿热和心脏病。

家族史无特殊。

体检：体温 36.7℃，脉搏 100 次/min，呼吸 20 次/min，血压 140/80mmHg（19~11kPa）。

发育正常，营养好。神志清楚，自动体位。无呼吸困难、发绀,无皮疹和皮肤紫癜,无浅淋巴结肿大。头颅及头部器官正常,颈软活动自如,无颈静脉曲张,气管居中,甲状腺不肿大。胸廓对称,肺清晰,心脏向左扩大,心律齐,心率 100 次 /min。心尖区闻及Ⅲ级粗糙吹风样收缩期杂音,无震颤,未闻及舒张期杂音。腹平软无压痛,肝于肋缘下 2 厘米处触及。肝颈回流阴性。脾未触及,腹部无移动性浊音。双踝微水肿,双膝反射活跃,无病理性神经反射。

X 线片:心脏广泛扩大

心电图所示:(1) 窦性心律

(2) 左心室肥厚

(3) 慢性冠状动脉供血不足

诊断:冠状动脉性心脏病

左室肥厚

心绞痛

签字:×××

日期:2017 年 5 月 13 日

Admission Notes

A 60-year-old married male was admitted on May 13, 2017, with a two-month palpitation and a thoracalgia.

Since this March, the patient has frequently felt palpitations and a chest pain upon physical exertion, the latter radiating into the left shoulder and arm. One attack lasts about five minutes. He has a feeling of suffocation. It seems as if something heavy were pressing hard on his chest. He has a slight cough and expectorates a little mucous sputum during the attack. Because he has not had any treatment before, the symptoms mentioned above have also deteriorated this week and his legs have been swollen as well, he came to the hospital for medical treatment.

During his illness, he has been feeling weak but he has had a good appetite, and his bowel motions and micturition have remained normal.

He said that he had been perfectly healthy and had never had rheumatic fever or heart trouble previously.

There is nothing particular in his family medical history.

PE T: 36.7 ℃ ; P: 100/min; R: 20/min; BP: 140/80mmHg (19~11kPa).

Well developed and nourished. In his right mind and in voluntary position. No dyspnea or cyanosis detected. No eruption or purpura over skin. Superficial lymph nodes impalpable. Skull and head organs not abnormal. Neck soft and supple and free of venous engorgement. Trachea in midline. Thyroid not enlarged. Chest symmetrical. Lungs clear. Heart enlarged and leftward without irregular beats. Heart rate 100/min. a grade−Ⅲ harsh blowing systolic murmur heard at the apical area with no thrill felt or diastolic murmur heard. Abdomen flat with no tenderness. Liver felt 2 cm below costal margin. Hepatojugular reflux negative. Spleen not palpable. No shifting dullness over abdomen heard. Slight edema in both ankles present. Bilateral knee jerk reflexes active. No pathological neural reflex found.

Chest fluoroscopy reveals general cardiac enlargement.

ECG shows:

(1) sinus rhythm

(2) left ventricular hypertrophy

(3) chronic coronary insufficiency

Diagnosis: Coronary Heart Disease

Left Ventricular Hypertrophy

Angina Pectoris

Signature: Dr. ... (M.D.)

Date: May 13, 2017

第二节 临床记录（Clinical notes）

1. 亚急性肝炎（Subacute hepatitis）

临 床 记 录

检查所见

男性　35 岁　　　6 英尺 6 英寸

无贫血

心血管系统　血压 120/85mmHg

心音 √

脉 56 次 /min,规律

胸部　　　　　√

腹部　　　　　√,但右季肋有轻压痛

Δ ?　　　　　亚急性肝炎

试验：肝功能试验

Clinical Notes

O/E

Male 35　　　6 ft 6 in

Not anaemic

CVS　　　　BP $\dfrac{120}{85}$ mmHg

Heart sounds √

P 56 reg

Chest	$\checkmark$
AS	Abd. $\checkmark$ apart from slight tenderness in R hypochondrium
Δ ?	Subacute hepatitis
	Reassure

Tests: Liver function tests

2. 胃病（Stomach trouble）

临 床 记 录

女性，29 岁

10 年前甲状腺功能亢进

胃病

情绪不好 1 年，服用地西泮。嗜睡

饭后 2~3 小时消化紊乱

食欲　　　差

体重 2016 年　　127 磅

　　　　2017 年　　113 磅

胃肠道　　便秘

月经　　　规律　　　　1 子（5 岁）

家庭　　　1 姐 +2 兄弟　健在

　　　　　父母　　　　　健在

体检

眼稍突出

眼外肌运动自如

无眼睑下垂或回缩

甲状腺可触及

右叶肿大 3 厘米 ×4 厘米

无杂音

无震颤

双手温暖干燥

心血管系统	脉	72 次 /min	规则
心脏	不扩大
心音	√
血压	120/80

呼吸系统　　　√

消化系统　　　√

中枢神经系统　反射未增强

足底反射↓↓

化验检查

促甲状腺激素（TSH）

血红蛋白

白细胞计数

红细胞沉降率

钡餐

胸部 X 线

颈部 X 线

Δ ?　溃疡病

? 　甲状腺功能亢进

? 　焦虑状态

Clinical Notes

Woman 29 years

Overactive thyroid 10 years ago

Stomach trouble

Depressed 1 yearr Valium. Sleepy

Dyspepsia 2/3 hours after food.

Appetite　　　Poor

Wt 2016　　　127 lb.

2017	113 lb.
Bowels	Constipated
Periods	Regular 1 son (5)
Family	1S+2B A & W
	Parents A & W

O/E

Rather staring eyes

EOM Full

No lid lag or retraction

Thyroid palpable

Ⓡ lobe enlarge 3 cm × 4 cm

No bruit

No tremor

Warm dry hands

CVS	P	72 reg
	Ht	not enlarged
	Ht sounds	√
	BP	120/80mmHg
RS		√
AS		√
CNS		Reflexes not exaggerated
		Plantar ↓ ↓

Investigations

TSH

Hb

WBC

ESR

Ba meal

C. XR

Neck XR

Δ? Peptic ulcer
? Thyrotoxicosis
? Anxiety state

3. 焦虑（Anxious）

临 床 记 录

检查所见
焦虑
心血管系　　　周围动脉脉搏 √
　　　　　　　脉 72 次 /min，规律
　　　　　　　血压 160/90mmHg
　　　　　　　心界不大
胸部　　　　　轻度肺气肿
　　　　　　　淋巴结不大
腹部　　　　　无肿物
中枢神经系统　无明显异常
Δ　　　　　　焦虑—安抚

Clinical Notes

O/E
Anxious
CVS　　　Peripheral pulses √
　　　　　P 72 reg
　　　　　BP 160/90mmHg
　　　　　Ht not enlarged
Chest:　　Slightly emphysematous
　　　　　No glands
Abd.　　　No masses

CNS NAD

Δ Anxiety—reassured

4. 计划生育（Family planning）

临 床 记 录

女性

结婚日期： 2006 年 4 月 12 日

妻子出生日期： 1985 年

初诊年龄： 30 岁

妻子职业： 家庭主妇

丈夫出生日期： 1982 年

丈夫职业： 劳工

生 育 史

年份	妊娠周期	存活情况	妊娠和分娩
2008	40 周	存活	顺利
2009	40 周	存活	顺利
2011	40 周	存活	顺利
2014	40 周	存活	顺利

一般病史

现在授乳： 否

头痛： 否

静脉曲张： 无

血栓性静脉炎： 无

黄疸： 无

过敏反应： 无

其他现在病症： 无

妇产科病史

最后一次月经：   2017 年 12 月 25 日

周期：   5/28

经量：   前 1~2 天较多

痛经：   无

白带：   无

盆腔感染：   无

性交障碍：   无

初诊检查

入口：   正常

阴道壁：   张力尚好

子宫：   前倾

子宫颈：   正常

附件：   正常

白带：   无

乳房：   √√

体重：   122 磅

血压：   120/80mmHg

2018 年 1 月 1 日   放置 DXW 77$\frac{1}{2}$ OJ

（Durex Watchspring 系子宫帽商品名，

77$\frac{1}{2}$为尺寸，Orthogynol Jelly 系杀精子

药膏）

2018 年 1 月 8 日复诊

Clinical Notes

Woman

Date of marriage: 4, 12, 2006

Wife's date of birth: 1985

Age at 1st visit: 30

Wife's occupation: Housewife

Husband's date of birth: 1982

Husband's occupation: labourer

Reproductive history

Year	Duration of pregnancy	Alive now	Pregnancy and delivered
2008	40	Yes	FIND
2009	40	Yes	FIND
2011	40	Yes	FIND
2014	40	Yes	FIND

General history

Lactating now: No

Headaches: No

Varicose veins: No

Thrombophlebitis: No

Jaundice: No

Allergy: No

Other current illnesses: Nil

Gynaecological history

LMP   25, 12, 2017

Cycle   5/28

Loss   Heavy 1st two days

Dysmenorrhoea: No

Discharge: No

Pelvic infection: No

Sexual difficulty: Satisfactory sex

Initial examination

Introitus: Normal
Vaginal walls: Satisfactory tone
Uterus: anteverted
Cervix: Healthy
Adnexa: clear
Discharge: Nil
Breasts: √√
Wt: 8 st 10 1b
BP   120/80mmHg

1.1.2018   Fitted DXW 77 $\frac{1}{2}$ OJ

                            (Durex Watchspring, size 77 $\frac{1}{2}$

                            OJ=Orthogynol jelly.)

See 8.1.2018

5. 产前检查（Antenatal examination）

临 床 记 录

女性 35 岁
妊娠——预产期 2017 年 7 月 10 日
一般状态尚好, 偶有疲乏无力
大便 1 次 / 天
无神经过敏或烦躁不安
无颤抖
无眼部症状

能较以前耐热

经常心悸

体格检查

健康妇女

心血管系统　　脉搏 88 次 /min，规律

　　　　　　　心界不扩大

　　　　　　　心音√

　　　　　　　血压 120/70mmHg

　　　　　　　胸部√

子宫近似足月妊娠。

舌苍白，无乳头。

颈柔软，甲状腺轻度肿大，无杂音，无震颤。

双手干燥、温暖。

中枢神经系统　反射√

　　　　　　　无眼部体征

Δ 正常甲状腺

? 贫血

Clinical Notes

Woman 35

Pregnant　　EDD 10.7.2017

Well but occ. c/o faintness

Bowels 1/day

Not nervous or jittery

No fidgets or shaking

No eye symptoms

Can tolerate heat better

Always had palpitations

O/E

Healthy woman

CVS   P 88—regular

                 Ht not enlarged

                 Ht sounds √

                 BP 120/70mmHg

Chest   √

near full term uterus.

Tongue pale and depapillated

Neck—soft and slightly enlarged thyroid. No bruit. No tremor.

Hands warm and dry.

CNS   Reflexes √

                 No eye signs

Δ Euthyroid

?   Anaemic

6. 血尿症(Hematuria)

<h1 align="center">临 床 记 录</h1>

四肢修长的健康女孩

无贫血症状

体格检查

心血管系统   脉搏 80 次 /min

                 心脏不大

                 心音√

                 血压 130/90mmHg

眼底   0

胸部   √

淋巴结不肿大

腹部   乙状结肠区轻度压痛

肾区无肿块

肛门指检　　　无异常
中枢神经系统　无异常

检查项目
IVP（静脉肾盂造影）
MSU（中段尿）
CXR（胸部 X 线）
FBC（全血细胞计数）
U and E（超声波检查）
RBS（随机血糖）

Clinical Notes

Thin long–limbed healthy girl

Not anaemic

O/E

CVS   P 80/min

           Heartt not enlarged

           Heart sounds $\sqrt{}$

           BP 130/90mmHg

Fundi   0

Chest $\sqrt{}$

No glands

Abd   Slight tenderness over sigmoid colon

No renal masses

PR   NAD

CNS   NAD

Investigations

IVP

MSU

CXR
FBC
U and E
RBS

7. 艾滋病（AIDS）

临 床 记 录

一般检查：鼻子和口腔周围有湿疹，口角干裂，左腋窝有一块面积 $10cm^2$ 的红色区域。除了头皮脂溢性皮炎外无其他皮疹。

血压：130/80mmHg

脉搏：90 次 /min

胸部正常

腹部无异常发现

在两侧颈部及两侧腹股沟发现软结节，其直径最大者达 1cm。

肛门周围发红，发炎? 疱疹性。

Clinical Notes

O/E   eczematous rash round nose and mouth/angular cheilosis.

Red area 10 cm^2 in L axilla.

No other rash except dandruff in scalp.

BP   130/80mmHg

P   90/min

Chest   clear

Abdomen NAD

Soft nodes up to 1 cm diameter both sides of neck and both groins.

Peri–anal skin: reddened, inflamed? herpetic

第三节 病情记载（Pathography）

1. 右膝关节肿（Swollen joint, right knee）

这是 1 例 15 岁男性病人，正舒适地躺着，没有急性病容，对时间、地点和人的定向力良好。血压 125/78mmHg，呼吸 20 次 /min，脉搏 84 次 /min，体温 102°（F）。心尖搏动最强点在左锁骨中线第五肋间。未触到震颤，心前区叩诊心脏不大。窦性心率、节律规则。仅在左侧第四肋间能听到往返性的摩擦音。心尖部有全收缩期柔软吹风样杂音，向腋下传导。主动脉瓣区第心二音大于肺动脉瓣区第心二音。胸部听诊和叩诊均正常。肝脏在右肋缘下一横指，无触痛。没有皮下结节或环形红斑。右膝关节发热、肿胀并有触痛。其他关节无疼痛，踝关节无水肿。

This is a 15−year−old male, who is resting comfortably, in no acute distress, and well oriented to time, place, and person. BP is 125/78 mmHg, respiration 20/min, pulse 84/min, temperature 102°. The PMI is at the fifth inter−space, left midclavicular line. There were no thrills palpated, and the precordium of the heart does not appear enlarged by percussion. The heart has regular sinus rate and rhythm. There is a to and fro friction rub heard just to the left of the fourth inter−space. There is a pansystolic soft−blowing apical murmur, which is transmitted to the axilla. A_2 is greater than P_2. The chest is clear to auscultation and percussion. The liver is down one finger's breadth below the right costal margin and is not tender. There are no subcutaneous nodules or erythema marginatum present. The right knee joint is warm, swollen, and tender to touch. There is no pain present over the other joints, and no ankle edema is present.

2. 前额痛（Frontal headaches）

威尔逊太太。她50岁了，5天来她前额部痛得很厉害，当情绪激动时多半就会发生，持续1~2个小时，休息或服阿司匹林都不能减轻。病人有5年的头痛病史，但是没有一次头痛像现在这么厉害。头痛不伴有恶心或呕吐，而且是间断发生的。2周来她的视力已经模糊。她不戴眼镜，以前也没有经历过这种情况。没有惊厥、晕厥或眩晕的既往史。她用力时确实有呼吸困难。没有胸痛、阵发性夜间呼吸困难、端坐呼吸或踝部水肿的病史。大约5年前，她因肾脏感染而治疗过。从那时以来，她曾有过多次的间断性的寒颤、发热、两侧脊肋角触痛和排尿时烧灼感，最近的一次发作是在一周以前。她母亲死于"高血压"，父亲死于"肾囊肿"。

Mrs. Wilson., who's fifty years old and has had severe frontal headaches for the past five days, coming on mostly when she gets nervous, lasting for one to two hours and not relieved by rest or aspirin. She has a history of headaches of five years' duration, but none as bad as the present ones. There is no nausea or vomiting associated with them, and they are sporadic in occurrence. Over the past two weeks she has had blurred vision. She does not wear glasses, nor has she previously experienced this condition. There is no past history of convulsions, syncope, or vertigo. She does have dyspnea on exertion. There is no history of chest pain, paroxysmal nocturnal dyspnea, orthopnea, or ankle edema. About five years ago she was treated for a kidney infection. Since that time she has had multiple sporadic episodes of chills, fever, bilateral costovertebral angle tenderness and burning on urination, the most recent episode being one week ago. Her mother died of "high blood pressure," and her father of "kidney cysts."

3. 左侧背痛（Left back pain）

病人到急症室前两天开始寒战、发热和咳嗽。出汗非常多并有左侧背部疼痛。是一种剧痛，他说："由于痛得我出不了气，所以我都不能呼吸了。"入院时体温是 103°（F），脉搏约 120 次/min，呼吸约 25 次/min。血压正常。

Two days before he came into the emergency room he began to have chills, fever, and a cough. He perspired profusely and had a pain in the left side of the back. It was a sharp pain, he said, "Cutting off my breath so I couldn't breathe." On admission his temperature was 103°, his pulse about 120 every minute, and his respiration about 25 every minute. His blood pressure was normal.

4. 胸痛（Chest pain）

这是 1 例 48 岁的男性患者。大约 2 周前，他开始感到乏力和食欲不振。2 天前的早晨，他感觉胸部有些疼痛，随深呼吸和咳嗽而加重。咳大量黄痰。整个白天一直是这种情况，当天夜里来到急症室检查。因诊断为肺炎而被收入院。

This is a 48-year-old man. About two weeks ago he began to feel weak and to lose his appetite. Two days ago, in the morning, he noticed some pain in his chest, increasing with deep breathing and with coughing. He brought up large amounts of yellowish sputum. He remained in this condition during the entire day, and that night he was seen in the emergency room. He was admitted with a diagnosis of pneumonia.

5. 弥散性甲状腺肿（Diffusely enlarged thyroid）

检查所见：体温 38.2℃，脉搏 82 次/min，呼吸 16 次/min，

血压 120/80mmHg。这个病人活泼健谈，并无急性的痛苦。无紫绀。皮肤有轻度红斑。头发：正常。眼睛：有点突出，眨眼次数较少，其他正常。耳鼻喉：正常。颈部：甲状腺呈弥散性肿大，比正常者大 2~3 倍，没有杂音。心脏：没有扩大，无杂音。主动脉瓣第二心音比肺动脉瓣第二心音稍强。窦性心律正常。肺部：支气管在胸正中线上。整个肺部的叩音呈高度反响，呼吸声微细。在双肺基底部有一些黏性啰音，无摩擦音可听到。腹部突出。吸气时肝脏从右肋缘降至 3 指宽处。脾脏：无法触知。右上腹部和腹上部有中度压痛。生殖器：正常。直肠指诊：前列腺Ⅱ度肥大。四肢：无浮肿。神经系统：肌肉运动极度衰弱与不协调。反应：对称而均匀，不呈病理反应，没有明显的感觉方面的缺陷。

P.E.T 38.2 ℃ , P 82/min, R 16/min, BP 120/80 mmHg. The patient was a talkative, alert, elderly male in no acute distress and without cyanosis. **Skin:** mild palmar erythema. **Hair:** not remarkable. **Eyes:** Slightly prominent, blinking somewhat infrequently, but otherwise normal. **E.N.T.:** normal. **Neck:** thyroid diffusely enlarged 2~3 times more than normal without bruit. **Heart:** not enlarged. No murmurs. A2 greater than P2. Normal sinus rhythm. **Lungs:** trachea in midline. Percussion note hyperresonant and breath sounds distant throughout. There were a few sticky rales at both lung bases; no rubs were heard. **Abdomen:** protuberant. **Liver:** descends 3 f. b. from right costal margin following inspiration. **Spleen:** not felt. Moderate R.U.Q. and epigastric tenderness. **Genitalia:** normal, Rectal: grade Ⅱ hypertrophy of prostate. **Extremities:** no edema. **Neurological:** minimal weakness and incoordination of muscle movement. Reflexes: symmetrical, equal without pathological responses. No definite sensory defects.

6. 阴道出血(Vaginal bleeding)

梅森太太 30 岁,第二胎第二产,她在妊娠期间一直来门诊检查。妊娠经过至今一直顺利,以前的妊娠也顺利。这是她目前妊娠经过的(简单)摘要。她的主要问题是 1 天前有阴道出血。出血量很多,需要用一整盒月经垫,甚至一条毛巾。出血是无痛性的,停止了几小时,接着又继续出血。病人是 36 周宫内妊娠。未入盆,无宫缩,未破水。目前未到临产期。听诊胎儿心音正常,每分钟 130 次。没有做阴道检查。血压 110/70mmHg,脉搏 100 次/min。还有轻度的心动过速。

Mrs. Mason is a thirty-year-old female para 2 gravida 2 who has been a clinic patient throughout her pregnancy. Her course has been uneventful up to now, and previous pregnancies were also without difficulty. Here is a brief summary of her present course to look at. Her major problem, as of one day ago, is vaginal bleeding. This has been profuse, requiring an entire box of pads and even a towel. It is painless, subsided for a few hours, and continued again. This is a thirty-six week intrauterine pregnancy. Not engaged, no contractions, and her membranes are intact. The patient is not in labor at present. Fetal heart sounds are well heard and are 130 per minute. A vaginal examination was not done. The patient's BP is 110/70mmHg, pulse 100 per minute. She also has a mild tachycardia.

7. 发热(Fever)

病人 15 岁,是第一次住院。大约在入院前 4 周,病人患了严重咽炎,伴有发热、头痛和呕吐,但没有皮疹。大约一周就好了,一直到住院前 2 天病人外表上看来健康。住院前两天他开始感觉有剧烈的心前区胸痛,吸气时加重,偶尔可转移到左肩。疼痛间断性发生,当病人向前屈身时可获得部分缓解。入院前一天,病人感觉右膝关节突然疼痛。该部位肿胀并有触痛。昨天开始发热,一直持续到入院。没有任何皮肤损害、不自主运动、厌食、体重减轻、鼻出血、气短或踝部水肿史。也没有眼眶周围水肿或血尿史。

The patient is 15 years old, and this is his first hospital admission. About four weeks prior to admission, the patient had a severe sore throat accompanied by fever, headache, and vomiting and was without a rash. This subsided in about one week, and apparently the patient was well until two days prior to admission, at which time he began to experience sharp precordial chest pain, which became worse on inspiration an occasionally would migrate to the left shoulder. The pain is sporadic in occurrence, and partial relief is obtained when the patient leans forward. One day prior to admission the patient experienced sudden joint pain in the right knee. The area was swollen and painful to touch. Fever began yesterday and persisted up to the time of admission. There is no history of any skin lesions, purposeless movements, anorexia, weight loss, epistaxis, shortness of breath, or ankle edema. There is also no history of periorbital edema nor hematuria.

8. 阴道分泌物异常（Bad discharge）

克拉克太太50岁,直到她来妇科门诊前大约1周身体还是健康的。这1周来她流出了一种黄绿色、带泡沫的阴道分泌物,伴有疼痛和排尿时烧灼感,并且在阴唇和阴道口周围有瘙痒。她在10年前已绝经了。经绝期后没有出过血,也没有腰背痛或骨盆痛。有过2次足月妊娠,2个孩子都健在。没有流产或早产史。1周来病人有点性交困难,这是她第一次碰到这种情况。病人有轻度肥胖,但没有高血压、多尿、烦渴或多食史。在体格检查方面,外生殖器出现明显的表皮脱落。阴毛分布正常。尿道口有显著充血。巴氏腺和尿道旁腺均无异常。阴道壁呈浅粉红色，无撕裂伤，但阴道内有黄绿色、带泡沫的分泌物。子宫颈居中并呈粉红色。宫颈口无梗阻，而其后唇有一个2cm×2cm大小的溃疡，没有明显出血。子宫和子宫附件均正常，直肠阴道检查没有阳性发现。

Mrs. Clark is fifty years old and was in good health up to about one week prior to coming to gynecology clinic. She has had a greenish-yellow, frothy discharge during this time, associated with pain and burning on urination and pruritus around the labia and introitus. Her last menstrual period was ten years ago. She has had no post-menopausal bleeding or pain in her back or pelvis. She has had two full term pregnancies and has two living children. No history of miscarriage or premature births. The patient has had some dyspareunia over the past week, and this is the first time she has ever experienced this. The patient is slightly obese, and there is no history of hypertension, polyuria, polydipsia, or polyphagia. In regard to the physical examination, the external genitalia appeared markedly excoriated. The hair distribution is within normal limits. The urethral orifice is markedly injected. Bartholin's and Skene's glands are not remarkable. The vaginal walls appear a pinkish white without any laceration, but with a yellowish-green, frothy fluid in the vagina. The cervix is in the midline and appears pink. The os is not obstructed, and there is a 2cm × 2cm ulceration not grossly hemorrhagic on the posterior lip. Uterus and adnexa are within normal limits, and the rectovaginal examination was without positive findings.

9. 肝硬化（Cirrhosis）

病人表现疲劳和营养不良。大体上说，他的肌肉组织显得消瘦。巩膜有轻度黄染。胸前有许多蜘蛛痣。皮肤也有轻度黄疸。腹部稍隆起,并有腹水。肝脏坚硬,边缘钝,在右侧肋缘下 5~6 指。还有脾脏肿大,腹部表面有明显的静脉曲张。踝部有轻微的水肿,并有肝掌。没有扑翼震颤。病人对时间、地点和人的定向力良好。隐血试验阳性。

The patient appears very fatigued and poorly nourished. Grossly, his muscle mass appears decreased. His sclerae are slightly icteric. There are numerous spider angiomata on the anterior aspect of the chest. His skin is also slightly jaundiced. His abdomen is slightly protuberant, and there is ascites. The liver is firm and the edge is blunt about five to six fingers below the right costal margin. There is also splenomegaly, and a venous pattern is evident over the anterior aspect of the abdomen. There is very slight ankle edema, and liver palms. There was no flapping tremor. The patient was apparently well-oriented to time, place, and person. Hematest was positive.

10. 胰腺炎（Pancreatitis）

这位 42 岁男性病人因主诉呕吐 3 天而第一次住院。每次呕吐之前都有恶心,3 天来每天呕吐 10~15 次。病人叙述呕吐物是白色、黏稠而不带血。病人喝酒有十多年了,3 天来他喝了大量的酒。在剑突下 7~8cm 处,他感到有一种钻孔样疼痛并向背部放射。这种疼痛还向右肩放射。没有寒战、发热或吃油腻食物后饱胀的病史。生命征均在正常范围内。病人表现非常焦急不安并很痛苦。对时间、地点和人的定向力良好。触诊时腹部有压痛,并在前述部位有自主性肌卫。肝脏在右肋缘下 4cm。肠鸣音稍减弱,没有板状腹。其余检查基本正常。

This is the first hospital admission for this 42-year-old male, who comes in with a chief complaint of vomiting of three days duration. He has had nausea before each episode, and has vomited ten to fifteen times per day over the past three days. The material has been described as whitish and thick and without blood. The patient has been a drinker over the past ten years and has been drinking quite heavily over the past three days. About seven to eight cm. below the xiphoid, he experienced a boring pain which goes through to the back. The pain also radiates to the right shoulder. No history of chills, fiver, or bloating after a greasy meal. The vital signs are within normal limits. The patient appears very anxious and in a great deal of pain. He is well-oriented as to time, place, and person. His abdomen is tender to palpation, and there is voluntary guarding over the area previously described. The liver is down 4 cm. below the right costal margin. Bowel sounds are slightly hypoactive, and the abdomen is not board-like. The rest of the examination is essentially within normal limits.

第四节　病史（历）（Medical history）

病史是病人病程记录的第一部分。它由六部分组成：主诉、现病史、过去史、家族史、社会史和系统复习（系统回顾）。在实际情况下，如果在几个方面为阴性，允许将几项合并或注明"无可记述"或"无关紧要"。

简单地说，主诉即患者就诊寻医的原因，可用患者的原话记述（用过去时态）；现病史是从医生的角度出发，对主诉进一步描述，比较全面完整；过去史包括过去的所有疾患、诊断、药物治疗以及免疫接种，还包括患者经历过的特殊事件及环境；家族史是记录患者的近亲（父母、兄弟姐妹、孩子）的疾病情况；社会史包括是否抽烟、喝酒，或有药物嗜好，以及个人旅游情况、职业和婚姻状况。系统复习是病史的最后一部分，是根据系统分类审查各种系统过去或现在的阳性发现。在这一部分，可按实际情况,只对个别有发现的系统加以陈述。

病史之前有统计资料（一般项目）,记录病人的姓名、年龄、性别及种族等。病史之后通常有"印象"一栏,是医生对疾病的初步诊断。

最后,写病史应基本掌握本专业内可能有的常用词（语）和表达法;在转述患者的话,即使用间接引语时一定要注意时态的转换。

1. 支气管哮喘（Bronchial asthma）

北京第一医院住院部

患者姓名：约翰逊
病 历 号：15672
出生日期：2010 年 6 月 4 日
出生地点：比利时、布鲁塞尔
性　　别：男
入院日期：2017 年 6 月 7 日

主诉：咳嗽,哮喘伴呼吸困难
现病史：

这是,该患者（7 岁,男）首次住院,他从 3 岁开始有哮喘病,但未因哮喘而住过院。入境后一直很好,入院前游长城出现气短,使用咳嗽药无效。哮喘逐渐加重,孩子被带到北京第一医院的急诊室,在那里接受肾上腺素和氧气治疗。然后,被送回希尔顿饭店。3 个小时后,孩子又被带回急诊室并收留入院。

过去史：

孩子 8 个半月出生。免疫接种：完全。过敏史：灰尘、洋葱。
家族史：

母亲 37 岁,健在。父亲 45 岁,健在。哥哥和妹妹身体健康。家族中无哮喘及糖尿病。

系统复习：

除有时有结膜炎及哮喘外，其他为阴性。

症断：

支气管哮喘

THE INPAIENT OFFICE OF BEIJING NUMBER ONE HOSPITAL

PATIENT' S NAME:	Johnson
CHART NUMBER:	15672
DATE OF BIRTH:	04/06/2010
PLACE OF BIRTH:	Brussels, Belgium
SEX:	Male
DATE OF ADMISSION:	07/06/2017

CHIEF COMPLAINT: Coughing, wheezing with difficult respiration.

PRESENT ILLNESS: This is the first admission for this seven-year-old boy with a history of asthma since the age of 3 who had never been hospitalized for asthma before. He had been perfectly well since he came to China until the touring the Great Wall prior to admission when the patient developed shortness of breath and was unresponsive to cough medicine. The wheezing progressed and the child was taken to the Emergency Room of Number One Hospital, Beijing, where the child was given epinephrine and oxygen. Then he was sent back to Hilton Hotel. The patient was brought back to the ER three hours later and was admitted.

PAST HISTORY: The child was a product of an eight and half month's gestation; Immunization: All; Allergies: dust and onions.

FAMILY HISTORY: The mother is 37, alive and well. The

father is 45, alive and well. One elder brother and one younger sister, are healthy. The family history was not positive for asthma and diabetes.

REVIEW OF SYSTEMS: Negative except for occasional conjunctivitis and asthma.

IMPRESSION: Bronchial asthma.

2. 清晨咳嗽（Early morning cough）

住院病人病历

一般项目：（省略）

主　　诉：约 10 年以来，每天清晨咳嗽，吐黄白色痰。

现　　症：病人是位 58 岁退休的工程师。他说患过慢性支气管炎，特征是约 10 年来，每天清晨咳嗽，吐黄白色的痰。由于这原因与膝关节炎，他在 8 年前退休。数月前开始咳嗽，这咳嗽与因支气管炎而起的咳嗽有些不同，它逐渐地严重了起来。这种咳嗽因抽烟（40 年来每天 1 包）而加剧，1 个月前病人停止抽烟。那时咳嗽似乎好了一些，但 3 星期前，他发现痰里有血。两星期前左胸部发生剧烈的刺痛。起初带有胸膜炎症状，后来有了 48 小时的胸膜炎性痛。自从那时起，除了胸臂运动与咳嗽时有剧烈刺痛外，疼痛慢慢地消失。在这两星期当中，他一直感觉微热，有些食欲不振和体重减少现象，但无恶寒。没有呼吸困难。据说住院那天所照的 X 光照片显示左肺中有一个卵圆形影，内有可疑的空洞。

既往史：一般健康情形良好。1979 年患过大叶性肺炎，1984 年患过病毒性肺炎。每次都有咳血。数个月前患病毒性肺炎但所摄胸部 X 线片显示正常。有一段时期他常患消化不良与腹上部疼痛，服用止痛片可缓解。否认有过肠胃障碍。30 年前患过肾绞痛，并且排出数个结石。以后没有再发作过。

家族史：母亲死于肺癌，一个妹妹死于结核病。其他正常。
妻子与4个子女均健在。

In-patient Case History

GD: (omitted)

CC: Early morning cough with whitish yellow sputum for about 10 years.

PI: This 58-year-old retired engineer stated that he had chronic bronchitis characterized by an early morning cough productive of whitish yellow sputum for about 10 years. Because of this and arthritis of the knees he retired 8 years ago. Several months ago, a cough somewhat different from that ascribed to bronchitis appeared and has become progressively worse. This cough got worse due to smoking cigarettes. (1 pack per day for 40 years), and he stopped smoking one month ago. The cough then seemed to have improved, but 3 weeks ago he noted blood-tinged sputum. Two weeks ago he developed a sharp stabbing pain in the left chest, at first somewhat but later actually pleuritic for a 48-hour period. Since that time the pain has gradually subsided except for sharp twinges associated with movement of chest wall or coughing. During this 2 week interval, he has had a low-grade fever, some anorexia, slight weight loss, but no chills. No dyspnea. Admission chest x-ray was said to show oval-shaped density with suspicious cavity in the left mid-lung field.

PH: General health is in good condition. Had lobar pneumonia in 1979, and virus pneumonia in 1984, each time with hemoptysis. A Chest x-ray made a few months after the virus pneumonia was said to be negative. He had recurrent episodes of indigestion with epigastric pain relieved by Pain Killer for a period of time, but denied other gastrointestinal complaints. Had renal colic and passed several stones 30 years ago with no recurrence.

FH: Mother died of lung cancer, a sister of tuberculosis. Others negative. His wife and 4 siblings are living and well.

3. 晚期乳腺癌（Advanced breast carcinoma）

晚期乳腺癌（右），轻度风湿性关节炎等（完全病历）

姓　　名：某太太

年　　龄：42 岁

性　　别：女

职　　业：家庭妇女

临时住址：罗蒂分克城市路 3 号

永久住址：波城公园路 35 号

婚姻状况：已婚

民　　族：克利尔

入院日期：2017 年 5 月 14 日

病历询问日期：2017 年 5 月 10 日

主诉：发现右乳硬结 10 年，急剧增大并发生溃疡 3 个月余。

现病史：9~10 年前，患者偶然发现右乳内有一硬结，黄豆粒大小、可活动、无痛，未予重视。硬结逐渐增大，但无不适感，生活劳动如常，故未就医。入院前两年前左右，肿块约已达 10cm×12cm 大。今年 2 月份起，迅速增大，越长越快，并觉疼痛，到上个月止，扩散至整个右乳，并发生溃疡，故来院治疗。近 10 年来大便不规则，每日 1~3 次，为黄色稀便，不带血和黏液，小便正常。食欲、睡眠尚好。近几个月来，体重约减轻 5kg。病程中无自感发热。

过去史：既往体健，幼年时曾患麻疹及腮腺炎，均于治疗后迅速痊愈，无结核及其他严重传染病接触史。

系统查询

呼吸系统：素有慢性轻咳史，多发生在天凉时，无午后低热、面颊潮红、盗汗及咳血史。

消化系统：童年时期常有腹痛发作及便虫史，药物驱虫后，发作性腹痛消失。曾有过上腹不适及右上腹疼痛，但无绞痛及皮肤、巩膜黄染史。无习惯性便秘或腹泻便秘交替史。

循环系统：偶尔有心悸及眼睑、颜面部浮肿，无呼吸困难、发绀史。重体力活动及上坡或跑步时，无明显不支情况。从无虚脱。去年 12 月至今年 2 月两小腿轻度浮肿，近 3 个月自然消失。从无淋巴管炎、淋巴结肿大及丹毒史。

泌尿系统：婚后曾发作一次尿急、尿频、尿痛。当时检查发现耻骨上区压痛，肾区叩痛阳性，诊断为急性膀胱炎，经治疗痊愈。无肾绞痛、血尿、脓尿及尿流中断史。

运动系统：患有轻度游走性关节炎，偶尔受寒后感全身疼痛。此外无骨、关节急性肿胀、疼痛、畸形及活动障碍史。

血液系统：无头昏眼花情况，无经常鼻出血或牙龈出血不止、瘀斑及轻伤后软组织严重肿胀等出血倾向史。

神经系统：近年间有前额痛史，经检查未发现严重疾病。无头昏、头痛、眩晕、麻木、瘫痪、感觉过敏、灼性疼痛及晕厥抽搐史。成年前生长、发育正常。第二性征明显。

手术史：因患右中指瘭疽，于 2006 年 5 月 20 日在莫延巴医院局麻切开引流，约 2 周后痊愈。

外伤史：记忆中无任何严重外伤。

个人史：出生于离此不远的一个乡村，曾于弗里敦短期居住过。未曾上过学。有吸烟及饮酒习惯，但均属一般。

月经及婚姻史：月经 $10\dfrac{2\sim3}{28\sim30}$，无痛经或经量过多、过少史。15 岁结婚，丈夫体健。婚后第五年初孕，孕 7，产 5，流产 2，平产 4，难产 1。现有 3 男 2 女，均健。

家族史：父亲患肺结核，长期慢性咳嗽、咳血，在患者幼年时期死于结核病。母亲死于衰老。外祖母于 1956 年 65 岁时死于子宫癌。此外，家族中无过敏史、家族性疾病及出血性疾病史。

社会史：患者系农村家庭妇女，与外界社会几乎无交往，从未远离家乡。否认卖淫及性病史。

以上病史系患者本人陈述，认为可靠。

体格检查

体温：37 ℃，脉搏：78 次/min，呼吸：22 次/min，血压：120/80mmHg（16/11kPa）。身高：1.60m，体重60kg。

一般情况：自然端坐，发育良好，营养中等，表情自然，神情合作，体态正常，步态自然，无异常活动。

皮肤：黑色，富有光泽，弹性良好，湿润度正常，无明显黄染，右中指近端指节桡掌侧有一约1.5cm长的萎缩性手术瘢痕。全身皮肤有散在性铜钱状癣。

淋巴结：右腋下可扪及多个大小不等质硬淋巴结，大者相互融合，不活动，右锁骨上窝及全身其他浅淋巴结均未触及。

头颅：发育正常，未见畸形。头发色泽如常、分布均匀。无炎症、水肿、旧瘢痕及压痛等异常。

面部：稍现苍白，但外观、气色正常。无压痛及水肿。无眼肌及面肌异常活动。

眼：双眉对称，无眉毛脱落缺损；眼裂对称，无睑下垂；双眼视力正常。睑缘无异常，结膜微红，无水肿，但有少量滤泡肥大及乳头状增生。眼球位置正常，向各方向运动自如，未见震颤及眼球突出；无巩膜黄染，角膜清透；瞳孔圆，大小对称，对光反射灵敏。视野及眼底正常。

耳：双耳廓大小及形状正常，无肿胀发红；双耳听力良好；外耳道未见耵聍及脓性分泌物；乳突无肿胀及压痛。

鼻：无鼻梁塌陷等异常，前庭正常，嗅觉良好。

口腔：唇红，无唇裂及口角歪斜，双侧鼻唇沟对称；舌红无苔，表面湿润，伸舌时无震颤及偏斜，齿龈颜色正常，未见齿龈萎缩及出血；口腔黏膜粉红，未见斑疹样损害，无龋齿，$\frac{6}{7}$缺损；腭及腭垂未见异常，咽峡正常，扁桃体不肿大，咽后壁轻度发红,未见淋巴结滤泡增生,亦无脓性分泌物附着。

颈部:颈软无畸形,甲状腺及唾液腺未见异常,气管居中,无瘢痕及淋巴结肿大,无静脉怒张及异常搏动。

胸部:胸廓左右对称,形状无异。双乳不对称,右乳肿块(详见外科情况),余无肿块及压痛。呼吸运动自如,对称。未见胸壁静脉扩张,亦无其他异常搏动。

心脏:

视:心尖搏动于左锁骨中线内第五肋间,未见心前区弥散性搏动。

触:触诊心尖搏动位置同上。未扪及震颤。

叩:心界测量如下:

右	肋间	左
0	2	0
0	3	3.0cm
0	4	5.5cm
0	5	8.5cm
	6	

注:前正中线锁骨中线间距离9.0cm。

心界无扩大。

听:心率78次/min,律齐,心搏强度正常,未闻杂音。桡动脉质地尚软,无异常脉律。

肺脏:

视:胸式呼吸存在,未见膈运动波。

触:语颤双侧对称。

叩:双肺野呈清音,无浊音及过度反响。

听:肺清晰,右下肺呼吸音减弱。未闻及啰音及摩擦音。

腹部:

视:腹平,无瘢痕,腹壁可见多条妊娠纹,无怒张静脉,未见肠型及肠蠕动波,腹式呼吸自如。双侧腹股沟无隆起。

触：腹软，无压痛及反跳痛，未触及质块及异常搏动；肝脾刚可扪及，质地中等，无触痛，双肾未触到，无振水波。

叩：无叩痛及移动性浊音。

听：肠鸣音存在，无减低或亢进。

脊柱、四肢：正常位置，无明显畸形，自主运动良好，无抽搐等异常活动，无触痛及肿块，肌张力正常，无皮肤及皮下异常增生、水肿、慢性溃疡及静脉曲张等征。指（趾）及指（趾）甲亦未见异常。

肛门、直肠：无肛周湿疹、肛裂、痔、瘘及肛周肿胀、压痛。括约肌张力正常。直肠内空虚，粘膜光滑，无肿块及阻塞。

外生殖器：阴毛分布正常，外阴已婚产型，无肿胀、水肿、压痛及白斑等，会阴未见陈旧撕裂征。

神经系统（反射）检查：

反射	右	左
二头肌反射	＋	＋
三头肌反射	＋	＋
腹壁反射	＋	＋
	＋　　　0	
	＋	＋
膝反射	＋	＋
踝反射	＋	＋
布鲁津斯基征	－	－
凯尔尼格征	－	－
巴宾斯基征	－	－

右乳外科情况：右侧乳房比左侧大，皮肤暗红色，呈橘皮样外观。右侧乳头抬高并回缩。外上限有一溃疡面，约3cm×3cm大小，溃疡中央有少量分泌物。右乳房内可扪及一肿块，约10cm×12cm大小，表面不平，质地坚硬，活动度极微，

明显压痛。右腋窝及胸大肌后可触及数个直径 1~3cm 大小不等硬淋巴结，大者表面不光滑，相互融合。

诊断:（1）右乳腺癌（晚期）

（2）乳腺癌转移至右腋淋巴结

（3）风湿性关节炎（轻）

（4）慢性支气管炎（轻）

（5）沙眼 I⁺（双）

医师签名：×××

病历写作日期：2017 年 5 月 20 日

Advanced Carcinoma of Right Breast, Mild Rheumatic Arthritis, Etc. (A Complete Case Record)

Name: Mrs. …

Age: 42 years old

Sex: Female

Occupation: Housewife

Temporary Address: 3 City Road, Rotifunk

Permanent Address: 35 Park Street, Bo

Marital States: Married

Nationality: Creole

Date of Admission: May 14, 2017

Date History Taken: May 10, 2017

Chief Complaint: The patient complained that there had been a hard protuberance over the right breast for ten years, rapidly increasing in size and accompanied by ulceration for over three months.

Present illness: About nine or ten years ago, the patient accidentally discovered a hard protuberance in her right breast, which was soybean—sized, moveable and painless, but she did not take it seriously. It grew slowly without causing any subjective ill effects. The patient did not seek medical treatment because she was able to live and work as usual. The lump had been about 10 cm × 12cm. in size some two years prior to her admission. Since this February, it had been rapidly increasing in size and growing faster and faster, causing pain. By last month, the lump had expanded to the whole right breast with ulceration. Therefore, the patient came to the hospital for medical treatment. In the last ten years, bowel movements had been loose and irregular, fluctuating between one and three times daily. Stools had been yellow but not stained with blood or mucus and urine had been normal. Sleep was rather normal and appetite fairly good but she had lost some 5 kg. in the last few months. During her illness, she experienced no subjective fever.

Past History: The patient was usually in good health in the past. She had measles and mumps in her childhood with quick recovery after treatment. No history was discovered of contact with TB or other major infectious diseases.

Review of Symptoms

Respiratory System: She usually had a slight chronic cough, especially in cold weather, but no history of low—grade afternoon fever, flushing, night sweat or haemoptysis.

Digestive System: Frequent attacks of abdominal pain occurred during her childhood accompanied by the passage of worms in her stools. These attacks subsided when worms were expelled with medication. Once she had epigastric distress and right upper abdominal pain, which was not colicky and was not accompanied by cutaneous or scleral jaundice. She had no history of habitual constipation or alternate diarrhea and constipation.

Circulatory System: She occasionally had palpitation and edema of the eyelids and face, but no dyspnea or cyanosis. During vigorous physical exercise, climbing hills or running, she felt no apparent failure of self—support and had never collapsed. From last December to this February, there was minimal edema of the lower extremities, which had disappeared spontaneously in the last three months. There was no history of lymphagitis, lymph node enlargement or erysipelas.

Urinary System: She once had an urgency and frequency of urination, and urodynia after she had got married. Tenderness over the suprapubic area and pain on percussion over the kidney area were found on examination performed at that time: the condition was diagnosed as acute cystisis, which was cured afterwards. She had no renal colic, haematuria, pyuria or pause in urine stream.

Musculoskeletal System: The patient had slight migrating arthritis, and occasionally had generalized somatalgia following chills, but otherwise she had no history of any acute swelling of pains, deformities or movement disturbance of bones or joints.

Blood System: She had no history of dizziness, vertigo, or bleeding tendencies such as constant epistaxis, prolonged gingival haemorrhage, ecchymosis or severe swelling of soft tissues caused by slight injury.

Nervous System: In recent years, she had occasionally had frontal headaches, but no serious diseases were found responsible for this through examination. She had no history of dizziness, headaches, vertigo, numbness, paralysis, hyperaesthesia, burning pain, fainting or convulsions. Before maturity, growth and development were normal for her age. Secondary sexual characteristics were obvious.

Operation History: Incision and drainage of infected right middle finger were performed under local anaesthesia in Moyamba Hospital on May 20, 2006. The wound healed about two weeks later.

Trauma history: She had no history of serious trauma as far as she could recall.

Personal History: The patient was born in a village not far from the hospital and lived in Freetown for a short time. She never went to school. She drank and smoked, but not heavily.

Menstrual and Marriage History: Her menarche started at the age of ten with periods of every twenty–eight to thirty days, lasting two to three days ($10 \frac{2\sim3}{28\sim30}$). She had no history of dysmenorrhea, hypermenorrhea or hypomenorrgea, and got married at fifteen. Her husband was in good health now. She had her first pregnancy in the fifth year of her marriage and had seven pregnancies altogether with five deliveries and two abortions. Of the five deliveries, four were eutocia (normal) and one was dystocia (difficult). Now she had three sons and two daughters who were all well.

Family History: Her father had pulmonary tuberculosis, a long–standing chronic cough and haemoptysis, and died of TB when she was a child. Her mother died of old age. The maternal grandmother died of hysterocarcinoma in 1956, at the age of sixty–five. Her family had no history of allergy, familial or haemorrhagic diseases.

Social History: The patient was a country housewife, had almost no contact with the outside community and never went far away from her home village. She denied either going whoring or contracting venereal disease.

The above history was stated by the patient herself and was considered reliable.

Physical Examination

T: 37℃ ; P: 78/min; R: 22/min; BP: 120/80 mmHg (16/11 kPa). Height: 1.60 m. Weight: 60 kg.

General Appearance: Natural good erect posture. Well developed. Moderately nourished. Natural facial expression. Clear and co-operative in mentality. Normal carriage. Natural gait. Normal body movement.

Skin: Black and lustrously rich. Good elasticity and normal moisture. No obvious jaundice. A contracted operative scar, some 1.5cm. in length, found on radial side of proximal phalanx of right middle finger. Scattered ringworms present on skin all over the body.

Lymph Node: Multiple lymph nodes, hard in consistency and varying in size palpable in right axilla with larger ones fused and immobile. No lymph nodes palpable in right supraclavicular fossa or in superficial areas of the body.

Head and Skull: Normally developed. No deformities observed. Hair normal in colour, luster and distribution. No inflammation, edema, old scars, tenderness or other abnormalities detected.

Face: Slightly pale without abnormal appearance or complexion. No tenderness or edema. No abnormal movements of ocular or facial muscles.

Eye: Eyebrows symmetrical without hair loss, epilation or damage. Palpebral fissures symmetrical without blepharoptosis. Visual acuity of both eyes normal. Palpebral margins normal. Conjunctivae reddish without edema, but with hypertrophy of a few follicles and papillary proliferation. Eyeballs normal in position with free movement in all directions. No nystagmus, exophthalmos or scleral jaundice. Cornea clear and transparent. Pupils round, symmetrical in size and acutely reactive to light. Field of vision and optic fundus normal.

Ear: Auricles normal in size and shape without swelling or redness. Hearing good in both ears and no wax or purulent discharge in external auditory canals. No swelling or tenderness over mastoids.

Nose: No saddle nose or other deformities. Vestibule normal. Sense of smell good.

Mouth Cavity: Lips red without cleft or corner deviation. Nasallip furrow symmetrical on both sides. Tongue red with moist surface and the absence of coating. No tremor or deviation on protrusion. Gingival normal in colour without atrophy or haemorrhage. Oral mucosa pink with no macula–like impairment. No caries. Left upper 6th and right lower 7th teeth absent. Palate, uvula and faux not abnormal. Tonsils not enlarged. Posterior pharyngeal wall slightly congested, but with no enlarged lymph follicles or purulent discharge.

Neck: Neck soft and supple without deformities. Thyroid and salivary glands not abnormal. Trachea located in mid–line. No scar or lymph node enlargement. No jugular vein prominence or abnormal pulsation.

Chest: Chest symmetrical and normal in shape. Breasts asymmetrical. A lump in right breast, which will be described under Surgical Condition. No mass or tenderness in the other. Natural and symmetrical chest movement with respirations. Neither venous distension of chest wall nor other abnormal pulsation observed.

Heart

Inspection: Apex beat seen in the 5th intercostal space, medial to left midclavicular line. No precordial diffuse impulse observed.

Palpation: On palpation, apex beat observed in the same location as on inspection. No thrill felt.

Percussion: On percussion, outline of cardiac borders measured as follows:

Right	Intercostal Space	Left
0	2	0
0	3	3.0cm.
0	4	5.5cm.
0	5	8.5cm.
	6	

Note: Distance between midsternal line and midclavicular is 9 cm.

Cardiac border not enlarged.

Auscultation: Heart beat 78/min. Rhythm not irregular, with normal intensity. No murmur audible. Radial pulse fairly soft in quality without abnormal rhythm.

Lungs:

Inspection: Thoracic respirations present. Phrenic wave absent.

Palpation: Tactile fremitus symmetrical on both sides.

Percussion: Lungs fields clear to percussion without dullness or hyperresonance.

Auscultation: Lungs clear. Breath sounds diminished over right lower lung. No rales or friction sound heard.

Abdomen

Inspection: Abdomen flat without scars. Pregnancy striae on abdominal wall observable. Dilated veins, intestinal patterns and peristaltic waves not observable. Abdominal respirations smooth. Protuberance of groins not present.

Palpation: Abdomen soft without tenderness or rebound tenderness. Masses and abnormal pulsation impalpable. Liver and spleen just palpable, moderate in consistency and painless on palpation. Kidney impalpable without sensation of fluctuation.

Percussion: No pain or shifting dullness to percussion.

Auscultation: Peristaltic sounds present without hypoperistalsis or hyperperistalsis.

Spine and Extremities: Normal in position without obvious deformities. Good for voluntary movement without abnormal manifestations, such as convulsions. No tenderness or masses. No abnormal muscular tension. No signs of cutaneous or subcutaneous abnormal proliferation, edema, chronic ulcer, varicose vein, etc. No abnormalities in fingers, toes, fingernails or toenails.

Anus and Rectum: No anal orificial eczema or anal fissure; no haemorrhoids, fistulae or circumanal swelling or tenderness. Tension of anal sphincter normal. Rectum empty. Mucosa smooth without mass or obstruction.

External Genitals: Distribution of pubic hair normal. Vulva being of married and multiparous type without swelling, edema, tenderness, leukoplakia, etc. No sign of old laceration of perineum.

Neurological (Reflex) Examination:

Reflexes	Right	Left
Biceps	+	+
Triceps	+	+
Abdominal	+	+
	+　　0	+
	+	+
Knee Jerk	+	+
Ankle	+	+
Brudzinskis	−	−
Kernigs	−	−
Babinskis	−	−

Surgical Condition of Right Breast: Right breast is bigger than the left. Skin dark red with appearance of orange peel. Nipple displaced upwards and retracted. An ulcerated area present over outer upper quadrant, approximately 3cm × 3cm. in size, with a small amount of inflammatory discharge in the center of ulcer. A mass, about 10cm × 12cm. in size, irregular on surface, hard in consistency, almost immobile and markedly tender palpated inside right breast. In right axilla and posterior to pectoralis major, a few hard lymph nodes varying in size from 1 to 3cm. in diameter felt with bigger ones irregular in outline, and fused together.

Diagnosis: (1) Carcinoma of Right Breast, Advanced Stage

(2) Metastasis of Breast Carcinoma to Right Axillary Lymph Nodes

(3) Rheumatic Arthritis, Mild

(4) Chronic Bronchitis, Mild

(5) Trachoma, Grade I$^+$ (Two Eyes)

Signature: Dr. … (M.D.)

Date　　May 20, 2017

4. 轻偏瘫（Hemiparesis）

住院病人病史

63 岁男性病人,因右侧轻偏瘫、语言构音欠佳为期约 5 个月,于 2016 年 12 月 11 日住院。

住院前 5 个月突感右下肢发麻无力,继而右上肢也有同样症状,神志清楚,无头痛。经当地医院治疗月余,症状有所好转,但直至此次住院时行动艰难,不能自穿外衣,言语模糊,发音不确切。

入院检查:神志清醒,体温 37℃。脉搏 80 次 /min。血压 180/80mmHg。头部五官无显著异常。颈部动脉博动对称,心律整齐,心率 80 次 /min,未闻病理性杂音。肺无异常体征。腹软。肝肋缘下刚可触及,质软。脾未触及。下肢不肿。眼底无视乳头水肿,有高血压性视网膜动脉硬化体征。神经病学体征表现右侧轻度中枢性颜面麻痹,舌伸出时往右偏,构音不清,无明显失语。右侧轻偏瘫,左侧肌力稍减弱,右侧腱反射增强。无明显半身感觉障碍。无脑膜刺激征。

实验室检查:血、尿、大便常规检查结果大致正常。血华氏反应阴性,红细胞沉降率第 1 小时末 16mm。空腹血糖 140~146mg/dl,饭后 2 个半小时血糖 231mg/dl。血清胆固醇 25mg/dl,β 脂蛋白 964mg/dl。血尿氮素 19mg/dl,CO_2 结合力

35.4 容积％。血清谷丙转氨酶（SGPT）50IU/L。TTT 和 TFT 结果正常。

其他检查：心电图：有冠状动脉供血不足征。脑电图：正常范围。脑扫描：正常。脑血流图：血管紧张度增高,搏动性和供血强度降低。颈椎及右肩 X 线片：有颈椎病和右肩关节周围炎征。

住院后应用中西药,包括复方丹参、抗栓丸（一种舒筋活血的丸剂）、活络丹、维生素 B_1、维生素 B_{12}、双嘧达莫、复方硝酸甘油、烟酸肌醇酯,以及根据血糖及血压具体情况使用适量盐酸苯乙双胍、复方降压片（双肼屈嗪与氢氯噻嗪）。另加用理疗、针灸等综合治疗。其症状明显好转,能自如行走,自穿外衣等,语言构音较前清楚。患者于 2017 年 1 月 25 日出院。

患者出院后在门诊治疗一阶段,至今症状平稳。

In-patient Case History

A 63-year-old male patient was admitted to this hospital on Dec 11, 2016 because of a right-sided hemiparesis and dysarthria of about 5 months' duration.

About 5 months prior to his admission the patient suddenly experienced numbness and weakness of his right lower limb. Subsequently he had similar symptoms with his right upper limb. He had no loss of consciousness or headache. His symptoms improved after receiving treatment in a local hospital for more than one mouth. He walked with difficulty, could not put on his overcoat, and spoke with indistinct or inexact pronunciation.

Examination on admission: He was conscious. Body temperature 37℃. Pulse rate 80/min. Blood pressure 180/80mm Hg. There was no significant abnormality in the head organs. The pulsations of the carotid arteries were symmetrical. The heart rhythm was regular.

The heart rate was 80/min. There were no audible murmurs. The lungs showed no abnormal signs. The abdomen was soft. The liver was palpable just below the costal margin and was soft. The spleen was not palpable. There was no edema of the lower limbs. The eye grounds showed no papilledema, but there were signs of hypertensive arteriosclerosis of the retinal arteries. Neurological examination showed signs of a rightside facial paresis of the central type. The tongue deviated to the right on protrusion. The pronunciation of speaking was not clear enough. There was no evident aphasia. There was a right–sided hemiparesis with slight muscular weakness on the left and increased tendon on the right. There was no definite hemihyposthesia. There was no sign of meningeal irritation.

Lab examination: Routine examinations of the blood, urine and stool showed essentially normal findings. Blood Wassermann reaction was negative. ESR 16mm at end of first hour. Fasting blood sugar 140–146mg/dl. Blood sugar 2 and half hours after meal 231mg/dl Serum cholesterol 251mg/dl β–lipoprotein 964mg/dl. BUN 19mg/dl. CO_2 combining power 35.4vol%. SGPT 50 IU/L. TTT and TFT normal.

Other examinations:

Electrocardiogram: Showing sign of coronary insufficiency.

Electroencephalogram: Normal.

Brain Scan: Normal.

Rheoencephalogram: Increased vascular tension with decreased pulsation and intensity of vascular supply.

X–ray films of cervical spine and right shoulder: Presence of sign of cervical spondylosis and periarthritis of the right shoulder.

After admission the patient was given both Chinese traditional medicines and Western drugs. These included composite Salvia Miltiornhizae preparation, Hacosan (a kind of antithrombotic vasodilator pills), traditional meridian activating pills, vitamin B_1, vitamin B_{12}, Persantin, composite nitroglycerine tablets, and inositol hexanicotinate tablets. He was also given appropriate dose of DBI tablets and composite hypotensive pills (dihydralazine and dihydrochlorothiazide), according to the values of his blood sugar and blood pressure. Besides, he received physiotherapy and acupuncture as a part of the combination treatment. His symptoms improved markedly in a few weeks' time. He was then able to walk around, to put on his overcoat by himself and to speak more clearly than before. He was discharged on Jan 25, 2017.

The patient had follow-up examination and treatment in the out-patient clinic. His condition remained relatively stable.

5. 股骨颈骨折(Femoral Neck Fracture)

病 历 摘 要

70 岁女病人于 2015 年 4 月 3 日因右侧股骨颈骨折入我院诊治。

入院检查:右髋部肿胀压疼,右下肢活动受限。X 线片显示右股头下部粉碎性骨折兼移位。建议行人工股骨头内修复置换术。经用药物及牵引治疗后症状减轻。患者要求回国进一步治疗。因而安排定于今日出院。

Medical History Abstracts

A 70-year-old lady was admitted to this hospital on April 3, 2015 because of having sustained a femoral neck fracture on the right side.

Examination on admission showed swelling and tenderness over the right hip. The movement of her right lower extremity was limited. X-ray film of her right hip showed evidence of a subcapital comminuted fracture of the femoral neck with displacement. An internal prosthetic replacement of the femoral head was advised. After application of traction and proper medication, her condition showed an improvement.

The patient had requested to go back to her home country for further treatment. It was, therefore, arranged that she be discharged today.

6. 急性胆囊炎（Acute cholecystitis）

住院病人病历

38 岁男性患者于 2017 年 7 月 11 日因右上腹疼 17 小时急诊入院。

患者于 2017 年 7 月 10 日晚饭后即感上腹疼，疼痛呈持续性并逐渐加重，向右肩胛部放射。呕吐 1 次。不觉发热。以往有数次类似发作。

入院时体格检查：神志清，痛苦病容。血压 140/90mmHg（1mmHg=0.133kPa）。脉率 84 次 /min。体温 38.5 ℃。巩膜无黄染。心肺正常。腹平坦，右上腹有明显压疼伴有肌紧张及反跳疼。肝下缘在右肋缘下 2cm 可触及。脾未触及。肠鸣音正常。

实验室检查：血红蛋白 160g/L。血白细胞计数 10 800/mm^3，中性多核白细胞 82%，淋巴细胞 16%，单核细胞 2%。出血时间 1 分 30 秒，凝血时间 30 秒。尿常规检查正常。血清淀粉酶 86 单位 %。血胆红质总量 1.3mg/dl，直接 0.5mg/dl。血清谷丙转氨酶、麝香草酚浊度试验及麝香草酚絮状反应皆正常。血尿素氮 12.2mg/dl。血二氧化碳结合力 55 容积 %。血型为 AB 型，血 Rh 因子阴性。

心电图正常。

超声波检查：右肋缘下近锁骨中线可见胆囊内液平面波（深 3.0~4.5cm），提示胆囊有增大。

胸部透视心肺正常。X 线腹部平片未见异常。

临床诊断：急性胆囊炎，可能并发胆石症。

入院后经禁食、静脉输液并滴注庆大霉素和硫酸新霉素，以及皮下注射阿托品等治疗，病人情况好转，腹痛逐渐减轻，18 小时后腹痛基本缓解，经医治 3 天后体温恢复正常。病人于 2017 年 7 月 18 日出院。

为了预防复发，建议回国以后作胆囊造影检查，并根据检查结果给予相应治疗。

In-patient Case History

A 38-year-old male patient was admitted on July 11, 2017 through our emergency clinic because of right upper abdominal pain for 17 hours' duration.

He stated to have the pain on July 10, 2017, soon after his supper. The pain was persistent in nature, gradually increased in severity and radiated to the right scapular region. He vomited once. No fever was noticed. He had similar attacks in the past.

Physical examination on admission: Mentally clear with distressing facial expression. Blood pressure 140/90 mmHg. Pulse rate 84 per minute. Body temperature 38.5℃. The sclera was not icteric. The heart and lungs were normal. The abdomen was flat with marked tenderness over the right upper quadrant, where muscular spasm and rebound tenderness were present. The liver was enlarged with its lower edge 2 cm. below the right costal margin. The spleen was not felt. The peristaltic sound was normal.

Laboratory examination. Hemoglobin 160g/L. White blood cell count 10 800/cu mm with a differential count of 82% neutrophils,

16% lymphocytes and 2% monocytes. Bleeding time 1 min. 30 sec. Coagulation time 30 sec. Routine examination of the urine was normal. Serum amylase 86 unit %. Blood bilirubin 1.3mg/dl with direct portion of 0.5mg/dl. SGPT, TTT and TFT were all normal. BUN 12.2mg/dl. CO_2 combining power 55 vol%. The blood group was AB and Rh factor negative.

ECG was normal.

Ultrasonic examination. Fluid waves of the gallbladder (at the depth of 3.0—4.5 cm) can be seen under the right costal margin along the mid-clavicular line, indicating enlargement of the gallbladder.

Fluoroscopy of the chest showed normal heart and lung. A plain film of the abdomen revealed nothing remarkable.

Clinical diagnosis: Acute cholecystitis with possible cholelithiasis.

After admission, he was put in fasting state. He was given intravenous glucose infusions together with intravenous administration of gentamycin, neumycin sulfate and hypo injection of atropine. His general condition was improved. The abdominal pain gradually reduced in intensity and was almost entirely relieved 18 hours after admission. The temperature returned to normal 3 days after the commencement of treatment. He was discharged from the hospital on July 18, 2017.

To avoid recurrent attacks later, it is advisable for him to have cholecystography done after he is back home and to receive further treatment accordingly.

7. 支气管肺炎、高血压、动脉硬化症（Bronchop-neumonia, hypertension and arteriosclerosis）

住院病人病历

病人，女，69 岁，因感冒后极度衰弱而于 2017 年 3 月 18 日至 26 日在本院住院治疗。

患者于入院前约 1 周感冒、发热，未得很好休息，病情逐渐加重。既往曾于 10 岁左右患小儿麻痹症。入院时全身情况差，极度虚弱，嗜睡，轻度呼吸困难。血压 180/100mmHg（1mmHg=0.133kPa）。心律齐。双肺底散在湿啰音。腹部胀气，检查欠满意。下肢轻度可凹性水肿。脊椎和胸廓明显畸形。血常规白细胞总数 19 200/mm³，中性白细胞 87%。K⁺3.2 mEq/L，Na⁺120 mEq/L，Cl⁻ 67 mEq/L。尿素氮 9mg/dl，二氧化碳结合力 97 容积%。血糖及尿常规检查正常。血液气体分析：pH 7.556，$PaCO_2$ 35.6 mmHg，BE+9.1mEq/L，SB 32.7mEq/L，AB 31.1mEq/L，PaO_2 70.1mmHg，$SatO_2$ 95.9%。胸部 X 线片示双肺稀疏散在斑片状阴影。

临床诊断：（1）肺部感染（支气管肺炎）；（2）电解质紊乱，代谢性碱中毒；（3）高血压动脉硬化性心脏病，完全性左束支传导阻滞；（4）肺源性心脏病待除外；（5）小儿麻痹后遗症。

入院后即予头孢菌素、新青Ⅱ号等抗菌素控制肺部感染；采用纠正电解质及酸碱平衡失调的措施；补充氨基酸和其他液体包括冻干血浆；继续口服地高辛 0.125mg，每日 1 次。经以上综合治疗，电解质紊乱有好转，但肺部感染及酸碱平衡失调情况尚未完全纠正。患者病情仍相当严重。建议留院进一步治疗。

In-patient Case History

A 69-year-old female patient was hospitalized in this hospital from March 18 to 26, 2017 because of severe general malaise following a cold.

The patient caught cold with fever about one week before her admission. She did not have a good rest. Her trouble became aggravated. She had contracted poliomyelitis in the past at about the age of 10. At the time of admission her general condition was poor, appearing very weak and drowsy with slight dyspnea. Her blood pressure was 180/110 mmHg, her heart rhythm was regular. Moist rales were audible scattering over the lung bases. The abdomen was distended with gas so that its examination was not so satisfactory. Both lower extremities showed mild pitting edema. Some evident deformities were noted over the spine and chest. Lab. Examination showed a white blood cell count of 19 200/cu. mm. with 87% neutrophils. Serum K was 3.2mEq/L, serum Na^+ 120 mEq/L and serum Cl^- 67 mEq/L. BUN was 9mg/dl and CO_2 combining power was 97 vol%. Blood sugar and routine urinalysis were within normal range. Blood gas analysis showed the following: pH 7.556, $PaCO_2$ 35.6mm.Hg. BE+9.1 mEq/L, SB 32.7 mEq/L, AB 31.1 mEq/L, PaO_2 70.1mmHg, $SatO_2$ 95.9%. X-ray film of the chest showed discrete, scattered, patchy shadows all over both lungs.

Clinical diagnoses: (1) Pulmonary infection (broncho-pneumonia); (2) Electrolyte disturbances with decompensated metabolic alkalosis; (3) Hypertensive and arteriosclerotic heart disease with complete left bundle branch block; (4) Pulmonary heart disease to be ruled out; and (5) Sequela of poliomyelitis.

After admission she was given Cefazolin and Oxacillin to control the pulmonary infection. Measures were taken to correct electrolyte and acid-base imbalance. She was also given aminoacid preparations and fluid with dry frozen human blood plasma. She was on oral digoxin 0.125 mg once a day. After such a combination treatment, her electrolyte imbalance improved, but her lung infection and acid-base imbalance were still not completely corrected. Her condition remained rather serious. It is preferable to have her continue staying in the hospital for further treatment.

8. 门诊病历（Out-patient case history）

【例1】

主诉：突发寒战，头痛、发热、咳嗽已有2天。

体检：体温 102.2 ℉。气色尚佳。咽部充血，扁桃体肿大。胸部和腹部阴性。

初步诊断：上呼吸道感染

治疗：青霉素 400 000 u.，肌肉注射，每日1次×3天（皮试后）

索米通1片，一日3次，连服2天

维生素 C，100mg，一日3次，连续3天，休息2天

签名　吴奇人

C.C.: A sudden onset wifh chills, fever, headache and cough for two days.

P.E.: T. 102.2℉. looks fair. Pharynx congested. Tonsils enlarged. Chest and abdomen negative.

Imp: U.R.L (upper respiration infection)

Rp: Penicillin 400 000u. (i. m.) q. d. ×3 days.(after intradermal test)

Somidon 1 tab. T. i. d. ×2 days.

Vit. C 100 mg. T. i. d. ×3 days. O/D (Off Duty)two days.

Signature:　Qiren Wu

【例2】

（男婴18个月）

主诉：发烧、咳嗽3天。昨晚恶化，出现呼吸困难，拒食。

今晨呕吐 1 次, 液状粪 3 次。（供史者：患儿母亲）

体检：体温：140 °F，脉搏：160 次/min，呼吸：60 次/min。苍白, 虚弱, 烦躁不安, 喘不过气来, 鼻翼抽搐。胸部：心跳规律, 但节奏快, 心音弱。肺部：两侧肺底可听到大量中等的和细小的湿啰音。腹部：柔软, 肋下 4cm 触及肝脏。未触及脾脏。

印象：支气管肺炎, 并发心力衰竭

治疗：（1）入院治疗

（2）吸氧

（3）青霉素 400 000u.（肌肉注射），一天 2 次（皮试后）

（4）链霉素 0.15mg, 肌肉注射, 一天 2 次

（5）西地兰 0.2mg, 肌肉注射, 立刻！此后 0.1mg, 肌肉注射, 6 小时 1 次, 2 次。

签字＿＿＿＿＿＿

(Boy, 18 Months Old)

C. C.: Fever and cough for 3 days. Became worse last night, with dyspnea appearing. The infant refused to suck bottle. He vomited once this morning, having passed liquid stools 3 times.

(Supplier of the Complaint: The Patient's Mother)

P. E.: T. 104 °F　P. 160/min.　R. 61/min

Looks pale and weak, restless and breathless with movement of the alae nasi.

Chest: Heart beats regular, but rapid and low. Lungs: A lot of small and middle moist rales on both lung bases.

Abdomen: Soft. Liver felt 4 cm below the costal margin. Spleen not felt.

Imp: Bronchopneumonia, complicated with heart failure

RP: (1) Admission

(2) Oxygen inhalation.

(3) Penicillin 400 000 u. (i. m.) b. i. d. (after intradermal test)

(4) Streptomycin 0.15 mg (i. m.) b. i. d.

(5) Cedilanid 0.2 (i. m.) Stat! And then 0.1 mg (i. m.) q. 6h. for 2 times.

Signature＿＿＿＿＿＿

【例 3】

姓名：王玉霞　　病卡号：W15–20835

性别：女　　籍贯：湖北武汉

年龄：31　　陈诉人：患者本人

民族：汉　　可信性：可信

职业：会计　　入院日期：2014.8.21.

婚否：未婚　　记录日期：2014.8.22.

地址：武昌洪山路 511 号

主诉：活动后心慌、气促，断断续续 2 年。心慌、气促加重，伴有阵发性夜间呼吸困难及下肢水肿 2 周。

现病史：病人 2009 年夏患过多发性膝、肘关节疼痛，伴有红肿，低烧，但无环形红斑样皮疹或皮下结节。经休息，服止痛药后渐愈，约 3 年无自觉症状，只偶尔感到两腿有点僵直。2011 年夏季起，渐感用力后心慌，气促，有时两下肢出现水肿。病人曾去社区医院就诊，诊断为风湿性心脏病。给予阿司匹林和激素，病情无好转，反而逐渐加重，体力减弱，休息时也常感心慌、气促，下肢水肿更明显。最近两周，病情进一步恶化，出现夜间阵发性呼吸困难、厌食、少尿。

过去史：无过敏史。有过童年期一般疾病。4 年前曾接受阑尾切除术。

家族史：父母健在，一个哥哥健在，无家族病史。

个人史：有少量社交性饮酒，不抽烟，无药物嗜好。

系统复习：如过去史

体格检查：

一般情况：T37.3℃，P 98/min，R 26/min，BP14/8kPa

患者发育良好，重病容，面色苍白，神志清醒，定向力好，合作；呼吸急促，唇部发绀。呈端坐呼吸体位。

皮肤及淋巴：皮肤平滑，无疹子或黄疸。右下腹部有 2 吋长、愈合好的手术瘢痕。表浅淋巴结未触及。

头部器官：无重要发现。

颈：颈软，气管居中，无结节或肿块发现。两侧静脉充盈，肝颈反流呈阳性，未见颈动脉搏动。

胸：两肺叩清。呼吸音略粗糙，两肺底部有少许细小湿啰音。正常女性乳房，无肿块或分泌物。

心脏：心尖冲动弥散，见于锁骨中线与腋前线之间、第 6 肋间隙处，心浊音界明显向两侧扩大，未触及震颤，心律齐，每分钟 100 次。第一心音减弱。心尖区听到Ⅲ级全收缩期吹风样杂音并向左腋部传导，三尖瓣区还可听到一低调雷鸣样舒张期杂音，未听到开瓣音及奔马律。在胸骨左缘第 2~3 肋间隙处听到另一舒张杂音。肺动脉第二音大于主动脉第二音。指甲床见到毛细血管搏动，臂动脉及股动脉处听到枪击音。

腹部：腹部平软，无腹胀。肝在肋下约 1.5 厘米处可触及，质较软，表面光滑，轻微触痛，脾未触及。

脊柱与四肢：脊椎正常。下肢，特别是踝部周围，有可见性凹陷性水肿。

神经系统和泌尿系统：无可记载。

实验室检查：

血常规：Hb110g/L，WBC6.7×10^9/L，N51%，L46%，E3%；

尿常规：蛋白（＋），WBC1~2/HPF，RBC10~12/HPF；

ASO<1:500；ESR2mm/h。

心电图：窦性心动过速，双侧心室肥厚，左心房扩大。

超声心动图：重度二尖瓣狭窄兼关闭不全及左房内壁有赘生物；中度主动脉关闭不全。

胸片：双侧心室肥厚及左心房中度扩大，肺纹理明显增加，提示肺充血。

印象:（1）风湿瓣膜性心脏病

（2）二尖瓣狭窄及关闭不全

（3）主动脉关闭不全

（4）双侧充血性心力衰竭

医师（签名）:＿＿＿＿＿＿＿＿

Name: Yuxia Wang

Sex: Female

Age: 31

Nationality: Han

Occupation: Accountant

Marital Status: Unmarried

Address: 511 Hongshan Road, Wuchang

Card Number:w15–20835

Native Place: Wuhan, Hubei Province

Informant: The Patient herself

Reliability: Reliable

Date of Admission: 08/21/2014

Date of Record: 08/22/2014

Chief Complaint: Exertional palpitation and dyspnea off and on for 2 years. Exacerbated above–described symptoms with edema over lower extremities and paroxysmal noctural dyspnea for the last 2 weeks

Present Illness: The patient had multiple pain in joints of the knees and elbows with low fever, redness and swelling in the summer of 2009, yet without erythema circinatum or subcutaneous nodules. It subsided after a period of rest and taking anodynes. For about 3 years, she was asymptomatic except for occasionally feeling somewhat stiff in the lower extremities. In the summer of 2011, she began to experience palpitation associated with exertional dyspnea as well as edema over the lower extremities at times In a local hospital her illness was diagnosed as "rheumatic heart disease". Aspirin and steroids were given, however, no obvious symptomatic relief was obtained, but her general condition gradually deteriorated, with dyspnea and palpitation occurring even at rest and aggravating, and more remarkable edema often occurred over the lower extremities.

Last two weeks, symptoms worsened further with paroxysmal noctural dyspnea, anorexia and oliguria.

Past History: No allergies. She had the usual childhood diseases. She was operated on for appendicitis 4 years ago.

Family History: Mother and father living and well. One elder brother alive and well.

No familial diseases.

Personal History: The patient has mild "social" alcoholic intake.

Review of Systems: As in Past History.

PHYSICAL EXAMINATION

General appearance: T 37.3℃ , P 98/min, R 26/min, BP 14/8kPa

The patient was well-developed, seriously ill and weak, with dyspneic and pale facial appearance and with cyanotic lips. She was in orthopneic position. She was alert, oriented and cooperative.

Skin and Lymph: The skin was smooth without any rashes or jaundice. There was a 2" well-healed surgical scar in the right lower quadrant of abdomen. Peripheral lymph nodes were not palpable.

Head: No important finding.

Neck: The neck was supple. The trachea was in midline. There were no nodes or masses present. The jugular veins were distended with positive sign of hepatojugular reflux; no visible carotid arterial pulsation.

Chest: Both lungs were resonant to percussion. Breath sounds were a little bit rough with fine moist rales over both lung bases. The breasts were normal female ones without masses or discharge.

Heart: a diffuse apical impulse was in the 6th intercostal space between the midclavicular line and the anterior axillary line, and the heart borders were unusually enlarged to both sides. No thrill was palpable. Cardiac rhythm was regular at 100 per minute. The 1st heart sound was in general poorly heard. A grade Ⅲ blowing pansystolic murmur radiating toward the left axilla and a low-pitched rumbling diastolic murmur were audible at the mitral area. No gallop sounds were heard. Mitral opening snap was not audible. Another diastolic murmur was audible in the 2nd and 3rd intercostal spaces along the left sternal border. $P_2 > A_2$, (The pulmonic second sound was louder than the aortic second sound). There was capillary pulsation of the nail beds. Pistol shot sounds were audible over the brachial and femoral arteries.

Abdomen: The abdomen was flat and soft without distention. The soft and smooth liver was palpable about 1.5 cm below the costal margin with mild tendeness. The spleen was not palpable.

Spine and extremities: Vertebrae were normal. Pitting edema was visible over the legs, especially around the ankles.

Neurological System and GU: Negative.

LABORATORY DATA

Blood Routine: Hb 110g/L, WBC 6.7×10^9/L, N51%, L 46%, E 3%.

Urine Routine: Protein (+), WBC 1-2/HPF and RBC 10-12/HPF.

ASO less than 1: 500; ESR 2 mm/h.

ECG: Sinus tachycardia with both left and right ventricular hypertrophy. Left atrial enlargement.

Echocardiogram: Severe degree of mitral stenosis and regurgitation with vegetations in the left ventricular wall. Moderate degree of aortic regurgitation.

Chest x-ray: Both the ventricles were hypertrophic and the left atrium was enlarged in moderate degree. The pulmonary vascular markings were remarkably exaggerated which indicated pulmonary vascular congestion.

Impression: 1) Rheumatic valvular heart disease

2) Mitral stenosis and insufficiency.

3) Aortic insuffciency

4) Bilateral congestive heart failure

Attending Physician (Signature)

第五节　病程记录（Progressive notes）

1. 大叶性肺炎（Lober pneumonia）

病 程 记 录

2017 年 5 月 3 日

患者本日入院，根据下列理由，作出大叶性肺炎的诊断：

（1）高热、咳嗽

（2）右上胸语颤略有增强

（3）右上胸闻及许多湿性啰音

（4）血常规：白细胞 21 000/mm^3，中性粒细胞 80%，淋巴细胞 19%，嗜酸性粒细胞 1%

（5）胸透：肺炎

治疗如下：

抗生素：青霉素 + 链霉素

对症治疗：喷托维林、复方阿司匹林等。

签字：×××

2017 年 5 月 5 日

入院后，患者自觉情况好转，已退热，咳嗽减轻，食欲增强。

体检：右上胸湿性啰音减少。

除链霉素停用外，其他治疗同上。

签字：×××

2017 年 5 月 7 日

患者感觉比前天更好,但有轻度咳嗽

体检:体温 37℃,一般可,右上胸仍可闻及少量湿性啰音。

白细胞:9 000/mm³,中性粒细胞:74%,淋巴细胞 6%

继续用青霉素。

签字:×××

2017 年 5 月 10 日

患者感到情况良好,不发热、不咳嗽,食欲良好。

体检:一般情况好,肺泡呼吸音正常,心音强、清晰而规则。

胸透:右上肺肺炎被吸收。

患者今日出院。

签字:×××

Progressive Notes

May 3, 2017

The patient was admitted to the hospital today with the establishment of the diagnosis of lober lobar pneumonia based on the following facts:

(1) The patient has a high fever, a cough productive of rusty sputum and a thoracalgia.

(2) Tactile fremitus is slightly deteriorated over the right upper chest.

(3) A lot of moist rales are heard over the right upper chest.

(4) Findings of routine blood test are: WBC 21 000/mm³, N 80%, L 19%, E 1%.

(5) Chest fluoroscopy reveals pneumonia.

Treatment given is as follows:

Antibiotics: Penicillin+Streptomycin

Symptomatiatria: Toclase, APC, etc.

Signature: Dr. ... M.D.

May 5, 2017

The patient has been feeling better since admission, her fever disappearing, her cough diminishing and her appetite improving.

PE: Moist rales over right upper chest have diminished.

The treatment given is the same as the above except that the administration of Streptomycin has been discontinued.

Signature: Dr. ... M.D.

May 7, 2017

The patient felt even better today than the day before yesterday, but still has a slight cough.

PE: T: 37℃. General condition fair. Some moist rales still heard over right upper chest.

WBC: 9 000/mm^3, N: 74%, L: 6%.

Penicillin continued.

Signature: Dr. ... M.D.

May 7, 2017

The patient feels all right, being free of either fever or cough and having a good appetite.

PE: General condition good. Vesicular breathing normalized. Heart sounds loud, clear and rhythmical.

Chest fluoroscopy: Pneumonia over right upper lung absorbed.

She was discharged from the hospital today.

Signature: Dr. ... M.D.

2. 泌尿道感染（Urinary Tract Infection）

病 程 记 录

　　4 岁女患儿，于 2016 年 10 月 1 日起经常反复发作泌尿道感染。

　　婴儿时期起，患儿即常患阴道炎。2016 年 10 月 1 日、2016 年 11 月 22 日及 2017 年 1 月 28 日曾 3 次患尿频、排尿困难和发热，尿常规检查尿蛋白均为（±），3 次尿沉渣内的白细胞分别为 8~12，6~8 和大量 / 高倍视野。患儿经用庆大霉素（第 1 次）、呋喃呾啶和复方新诺明治疗后迅速好转。

　　患儿于 2017 年 4 月 9 日，继发热及上呼吸道感染，第 4 次发作尿道炎。查尿：蛋白（-），沉渣内白细胞 11~13/ 高倍视野。通常治疗不能控制感染。多次尿沉渣仍有白细胞 5~8/ 高倍视野，使用萘丁酸治疗 2 周后，尿检正常。建议继续应用呋喃丹啶 3 个月。

　　尿培养检查结果如下：2017 年 2 月 21 日有大肠杆菌、副大肠杆菌和肠球菌生长。细菌计数为 4 800/ml。2017 年 3 月 1 日有大肠杆菌和副大肠杆菌生长。细菌计数为 15 400/ml。2017 年 5 月 3 日末梢白细胞计数为 5 200/mm^3，分类为中性粒细胞 42%、淋巴细胞 51%、嗜酸粒细胞 1%、单核 6%。

　　由于患儿有反复发作的泌尿道感染病史，第 4 次发作时治疗又不够顺利，建议进一步做静脉肾盂造影（排泄性尿路造影）以除外先天性泌尿畸形的可能性。

Progressive Notes

A 4-year-old girl has had recurrent urinary tract infections since Oct 1, 2016.

She has had frequent attacks of vaginitis since infancy. She had three attacks of frequency of urination, dysuria and fever on Oct 1,

2016, Nov 22, 2016 and Jan 28, 2017.Urine examinations revealed the following: Albumin (±), white blood cells were found to be 8~12, 6~8 and numerous/HPF on 3 occasions in the urine sediment. She improved quickly on gentamycin (during the first attack), nitrofuradantin and SMZ plus TMP treatments.

She had the fourth attack on April 9, 2017 following fever and upper respiratory track infection. Urine examination revealed the following: albumin (−), white blood cells 11~13/HPF in the sediment. The infection could not be controlled with the usual treatment and there were WBC 5~8/HPF in the urine sediment on several occasions. She received nalidixic acid treatment for two weeks, then the urine was normal. She was advised to keep on nitrofuradantin treatment for three months.

Urine culture on Feb 21, 2017 grew B. coli, B. coli communior and Streptococcus fecalis, bacterial count being 4 800/ml, another urine culture on March 1, 2017 grew B. coli and B. coli communior, bacterial count being 15 400/ml. White blood cell count (peripheral blood) on May 3, 2017 revealed a total count of 5 200/cu. mm. With a differential count as follows: Neutrophils 42%, lymph 51%, eosin 1%, and mono 6%.

On account of her history of recurrent urinary tract infections, with the fourth attack relatively resistant to treatment, intravenous pyelography with excretory urography is advised to rule out the possibility of any congenital anomalities in the urinary tract.

3. 腰椎结核（**TB of Lumbar Spine**）

病 程 记 录

26 岁女病人于 2014 年 8 月因腰疼 1 月余，在我院就诊。X 线腰椎照相检查发现第 1、2 腰椎体明显破坏，腰椎表现局部轻度后突畸形，此外并有双侧腰大肌脓肿形成征象，遂于 2014 年 9 月 23 日住院治疗。

入院时患者体温 37.5~38℃。营养状况差，消瘦，第一腰椎处脊椎后突畸形，局部有压疼，腰部活动受限。

入院后检查：红细胞沉降率增快，曾高达 86mm/第 1 小时末（韦氏法）。

经数月卧石膏床休息，症状稳定，于 2015 年 2 月 27 日在硬脊膜外麻醉下行腰椎结核灶清除术。同时作了腰大肌寒性脓肿引流术，髂骨取骨和第 1、2 腰椎椎体间植骨术。术后继续抗结核治疗，并卧床休养半年。2015 年 10 月 25 日出院。全身情况明显改进。

出院后继续在我院门诊随诊。红细胞沉降率恢复正常。

2016 年 11 月 28 日腰椎 X 线照像显示椎体间植骨片已呈骨性愈合。

Progressive Notes

A 26-year-old woman patient was seen in our out-patient clinic in August, 2014, because of lumbar pain of more than one month's duration. X-ray examination of her lumbar spine showed evidence of destructive lesions of the bodies of the 1st or 2nd lumbar vertebrae with local, slightly kyphotic deformity and signs of bilateral psoas abscesses. She was then admitted on Sept 23, 2014 for treatment.

After admission she was found to have a body temperature of 37.5-38.0℃. She appeared to be with a fairly poor nutritional status. There was a gibbous deformity at the level of the first lumbar vertebra with local tenderness and limitation of the lumbar movements.

Examination after admission showed that her ESR was increased, rising up to 86 mm at the end of the first hour (by Westergren method).

After a few months' rest in a plaster bed, her symptoms became stable. On Feb. 27, 2015, under extradural anaesthesia excision of the tuberculous foci of the lumbar spine was performed together with drainage of the psoas cold abscesses and intervertebral bone grafting between the bodies of the 1st and 2nd lumbar vertebrae, using an autograft taken from the ilium. Postoperatively the patient continued to be on anti-tuberculosis therapy and lay in bed for half a year for her convalescence. She was discharged on Oct. 25, 2015 with marked improvement of her general condition.

The patient continued to have follow-up examinations in our out-patient clinic. The ESR returned to normal.

X-ray re-examination of her lumbar spine on Nov. 28, 2016 showed that the intervertebral bone graft healed with bony union.

4. 骨软骨瘤（Osteochondroma）

病 程 记 录

25 岁男病人因右股骨远端外侧无痛肿物,伴有轻度右膝不适感于 2015 年 11 月 17 日入院。入院临床诊断为右股骨骨软骨瘤。

住院后于 2015 年 11 月 24 日切除约 2cm 直径大小骨软骨瘤。病理检查结果证实临床诊断。2015 年 12 月 4 日行尿道外口乳头状肿物活体检查和电烙术。病理检查证实为乳头状瘤。

术后恢复顺利。患者于 2015 年 12 月 6 日出院。建议出院后应定期随诊。

Progressive Notes

A 25-year old male patient was admitting to our hospital on Nov 17, 2015, because of a bulging, painless mass on the lateral aspect of the distal end of the right femur, with slight discomfort of the right knee. The clinical diagnosis on admission was osteochondroma of the right femur.

An operation was performed on Nov. 24, 2015. An osteochondroma of about 2 cm in diameter was removed. The clinical diagnosis was verified by the result of the pathological examination.

On Dec. 4, 2015 biopsy and electrocautery were done to remove the papillary tumor of the external urethral orifice. It was shown to be a papilloma on pathological examination.

The postoperative course was uneventful. He was discharged on Dec. 6, 2015.He was advised to have follow-up examinations after his discharge at regular intervals.

5. 急性肺炎（Acute pneumonia）

病　程　记　录

25 岁女病人因发热、咳嗽 3 天于 2017 年 7 月 11 日住入医院。

入院查体：体温 39.8℃。轻度呼吸困难。右后下胸部叩诊有浊音，听诊于吸气末可闻湿啰音。X 线胸部正位片可见右下肺野斑片状模糊阴影，侧位片可见于右下叶后基底段和中叶。血白细胞计数为 14 000/mm³，其中中性分叶核细胞占 86%。临床诊断为右中、下叶急性肺炎。

住院后给予庆大霉素 8 万单位，一日 2 次，肌内注射；水剂青霉素 G 80 万单位，一日 3 次，肌肉注射。患者体温在 3 天内降至正常，肺部情况明显好转。患者于 2017 年 7 月 17 日出院。

建议出院后口服氨基苄青霉素 0.5g，一日 4 次，连服 3 天；氨茶碱 0.1g，一日 3 次；溴己新 16mg，一日 3 次。并建议定期在当地医院继续复查处理。

Progressive Notes

A 25-year-old lady was admitted to this hospital on July 11, 2017 because of fever and cough of 3 days' duration.

Physical examination on admission. Body temperature 39.8℃. She was found to be slightly dyspnea. The right lower posterior chest showed dullness on percussion, with moist rales at the end of inspiration on ausucltation. X-ray films of the chest showed cloudy patches over the right lower lung field in the posterior-anterior view and over the postero-basal segment of the right lower lobe and the right middle lobe in the lateral view. The white blood cell count was 14 000 per cu mm with a 86% of polymorphonuclear neutrophils in the differential count. The clinical diagnosis was acute pneumonia involving the right middle and lower lobes.

After admission she was given Gentamycin 80 000 units intramuscularly twice a day and Penicillin G 800 000 units intramuscularly three times a day. Her body temperature dropped to normal within three days and her lung condition improved markedly. She was discharged on July 17, 2017.

After her discharge, she is advised to take ampicillin 0.5g orally four times a day for three successive days, aminophylline 0.1g three times a day and bisolvon (bromhexine) 16mg three times a day. She is also advised to have further examinations and treatment at intervals in a local hospital.

6. 左下肺肺炎（Pneumonia, Left lower lung）

病 程 记 录

75 岁女病人因咳嗽 4 天, 发冷发热伴铁锈色痰 1 天, 于 2017 年 3 月 20 日至 3 月 26 日住院诊治。

入院时体温38.4℃,血压100/60mmHg。化验血白细胞14 000~21 000/mm³,中性白细胞91%。胸部X线片示肺纹理增厚,左下肺心缘可见片状模糊阴影。心脏呈主动脉型,主动脉曲屈延长。痰培养肺炎双球菌生长。尿常规、肝功能、肾功能等检查正常。

住院后即予青霉素、庆大霉素及止咳祛痰药治疗。体温逐渐下降。入院后第三天起改用红霉素,复方三甲氧苄氨嘧啶片口服,临床症状明显好转,体力恢复。根据患者旅行安排,同意近期出院。

出院建议:避免劳累,受凉;按医嘱服药,到医院复查。

临床诊断:左下肺肺炎。

Progressive Notes

A 75-year-old lady was hospitalized in this hospital from March 20 to 26, 2017 because of having coughed for four days with rusted sputum on top of chills and fever of one day's duration.

On admission her body temperature was 38.4℃ , and her blood pressure 100/60mm Hg. Laboratory examination showed white blood cell counts varied from 21 000 to 14 000/cu mm with 91% neutrophils. X-ray film of the chest showed increased lung markings with a patch of hazy shadow in the left lower lung near the heart border. The heart appeared to be of aortic type with a tortuous and prolonged aorta.

Culture of the sputum showed growth of streptococcus pneumoniae. Routine urinalysis and tests of the liver and kidney functions showed normal findings.

After admission she was treated with penicillin G, gentamycin and anti-cough drugs together with expectorants. The body temperature was dropping gradually. Beginning from the third day on,

Erythromycin and Tablet TMP Co. were administered orally instead. The clinical symptoms improved markedly with increase of her body strength. It was agreed that in keeping with her travelling schedule she will be discharged pretty soon. It is advised that after discharge she should avoid over-fatigue and cold, take the medication as directed by the physician in charge, and have follow-up observation in a hospital.

Clinical Diagnosis: Pneumonia, left lower lung

第六节　手术记录（Operative notes）

1. 阑尾切除术（Appendectomy）（例1）

手 术 记 录

姓名：某先生

手术日期：2017 年 11 月 17 日

术前诊断：急性化脓性阑尾炎、局限性腹膜炎

手术名称：阑尾切除术

术后诊断：同术前诊断

手术者：×××医师

麻醉：硬膜外麻醉

麻醉师：×××医师

手术步骤：硬膜外麻醉后，患者取仰卧位。术野用碘酒及酒精常规消毒，覆盖手术单。

作麦氏切口，约 8cm 长。切开皮肤及皮下组织，钳夹出血点，丝线结扎止血。循纤维方向剪开腹外斜肌筋膜，切开肌膜后，在肌肉上作一小切口，用一把直钳行钝性分离，用手指剥离肌肉并牵开直达腹膜。而后切开腹膜进入腹腔，盲肠及阑尾便

显现于术野。助手用左手上的湿纱布提起盲肠，阑尾便从伤口中显露出来。以一把鼠齿钳夹住阑尾尖端系膜并提起阑尾。分次钳夹、切断、结扎阑尾系膜，双层结扎阑尾动脉，钳夹阑尾基底部，然后用肠线牢固结扎。以 4 号线绕阑尾基底的盲肠壁作浆肌层的荷包缝合，周围用一块纱布保护以免污染。距阑尾基部约 0.5cm 处切断阑尾并取出，残端涂抹碘酒、苯酚和酒精。逐渐收紧荷包缝合，以细长钳子夹住阑尾的结扎线，并内推，最后收紧荷包缝合，包埋阑尾残端。

　　关腹前，检查结扎后的阑尾系膜正常，未见出血。核对器械和敷料数，与术前无误。用生理盐水冲洗局部腹腔并吸尽，分层缝合腹壁。麻醉满意。术中失血 10~30ml。手术顺利，术中患者情况良好，手术后患者被送到病房。

Operative Notes

Name: Mr. …

Date of Operation: November 17, 2017

Preoperative Diagnosis: Acute Purulent Appendicitis and Localized Peritonitis

Name of Operation: Appendectomy

Postoperative Diagnosis: The Same as Above

Operator: Dr. …

Anaesthesia: Epidural

Anaesthetist: Dr. …

Procedure: The patient was placed in the dorsal position after epidural anaesthesia. The field of operation was routinely prepared with tincture of iodine, and alcohol and then the patient was draped with sterile abdominal sheets.

A Mcburneys incision was made, approximately 8cm. The skin and subcutaneous tissue were incised, bleeding points clamped and tied with silk to control bleeding. The fascia of the external oblique muscle was cut with scissors along its muscular fibres. With the incision of the muscle fascia, a small opening was made in the muscles by blunt dissection performed with a pair of straight forceps; the muscles were split with fingers and retracted towards both sides till the peritoneum was reached. The peritoneum was subsequently incised and access to the abdominal cavity gained, the cecum and appendix presented in the field of operation. The cecum was elevated with a moist pack by the left hand of the assistant, the appendix delivered out of the wound. The mesoappendix was held taut at its tip and the appendix elevated with a pair of Allis forceps. The mesoappendix was clamped, severed and suture–ligated in sections and the appendicular artery doubly suture–ligated. The base of the appendix was tightly crushed and a tight ligature tied with catgut around the crushed area. A purse–string suture passing through the serous and muscular layers of the cecum wall around the base of the appendix was made with silk No. 4 and it was protected from contamination all around with a piece of gauze. The appendix was severed 0.5cm. from the appendicular base and taken out, with the stump of the appendix treated in succession with tincture of iodine, carbolic acid and alcohol. While the purse–string suture was gradually tightened, the appendicular stump was invaginated with the aid of fine–tipped forceps applied to the ligature on the stump. Finally, the purse–string suture was completely tightened with the stump carefully embedded within it.

Before the abdomen was closed, the ligatured mesoappendix was re–examined and found normal and free of bleeding. Instruments and gauze pads were counted and their numbers found identical with the ones on the preoperative list. The area of the abdominal cavity was washed with NS. All the fluid was removed by suction.

The abdominal wall was sutured in layers. About 10~30 ml of blood was lost during the operation. With satisfactory anaesthesia, the patient's vital signs remained normal throughout the operation, which was uneventful. The patient was taken back to the ward after the operation.

2. 阑尾切除术（Appendectomy）（例 2）

手术记录

术前诊断：急性阑尾炎

术后诊断：急性阑尾炎

已施手术：阑尾切除

手术步骤：病员取仰卧位，腹壁用碘酒和酒精消毒后铺上消毒巾，局麻后作麦氏切口，所有出血点均用细丝线结扎止血。进入腹腔时未见脓液。阑尾位于回盲部，长约 8cm，直径 0.8cm。显著充血水肿，其尖端埋入渗出物中，然而其基部大致正常。

其他所见脏器包括部分盲肠、升结肠和回肠均正常，伤口边缘用湿纱布垫隔开，游离阑尾后，在阑尾系膜上夹一把血管钳，阑尾系膜在血管钳之间切断直至基底部。系膜血管用中丝线双重结扎，在盲肠的阑尾根部周围用细丝线作一荷包缝合。阑尾根部经挤压后用粗丝线结扎，周围用湿纱布隔开，在结扎远侧 0.3cm 处切除阑尾。然后阑尾残端依次用浸泡过石炭酸、95% 乙醇和 0.9% 氯化钠溶液的棉拭子涂擦，并将其置之荷包缝使之内翻。除去保护用的盐水纱布，将盲肠回纳腹腔，检查有无出血点和异物后，伤口用 0.9% 氯化钠溶液冲洗，并按需要用 00 号铬质肠线和丝线分层缝合。手术过程平稳，病员送回病房，情况良好。

未予输血，未行引流，标本已送病理检查。

Operative Notes

Preoperative diagnosis: Acute appendicitis

Postoperative diagnosis: Acute appendicitis

Operation: Appendectomy

Procedure: With the patient in the supine position, the abdominal wall was prepared with tincture iodine and alcohol and draped. Under local anesthesia, a McBurney's incision was made. All bleeders were clamped and tied with fine silk. When the abdominal cavity was entered, no pus was found. The appendix was situated in the ilio–cecal region. It was about 8 cm in length and 0.8 cm in diameter. It was very much congested and edematous with its tip embedded in the exudate, its base being apparently normal.

The remaining viscera seen, including part of the cecum, the ascending colon, and the terminal ileum, all appeared normal. The wound edges were walled off with wet packs. After delivering the appendix, a clamp was placed on its mesentery near the tip. The mesentery of the appendix was divided between clamps down to the base. The mesenteric vessels were double tied with medium silk. A fine silk purse–string suture was next placed in the cecum around the base of the appendix. The base was crushed and a heavy silk tie was then applied. The area was then walled off with a wet sponge and the appendix was amputated just 0.3cm distal to the tie. The stump of the appendix was touched in succession with swabs dipped in phenol, 95% alcohol and normal saline, and was inverted by the purse–string already placed. The protecting saline sponge was then removed and discarded. The cecum was put back into the abdominal cavity. After having looked for bleeders and foreign bodies, the wound was irrigated with normal saline and closed in layers with No. 00 chromic catgut and silk accordingly. The course of the operation was smooth and the patient was sent back to the ward in good condition.

No blood transfusion and no drain employed. The specimen was sent for pathological examination.

第七节　专用证明（Special certificate）

1. 死亡证明（Certificate of death）

死 亡 证 明

58 岁男性患者于 2016 年 6 月 30 日晨突然死亡送往我院急诊室。

患者于晨 7 时 50 分在其旅馆餐厅内突然摔倒。当医生马上来诊视时已不见心跳或呼吸。遂施以人工呼吸与体外心脏按压并送我院做进一步抢救。患者于晨 9 时抵达急救室时均不见心跳、呼吸。经持续抢救达 40 分钟,包括采用心脏按压、人工吸氧、心肌内注射肾上腺素及异丙基肾上腺素等措施均归无效。

据其代表团其他成员反映,既往有心脏病及心律失常病史。

诊断:心源性猝死。

抢救时其夫人在场。经其使馆申请,遗体于同日作防腐处理。

Certificate of Death

A 58-year-old male was sent to the emergency clinic of our hospital because of sudden death in the morning of June 30, 2016.

He fell down in the dining room of his hotel at 7: 50 a.m. and no heart beat nor respiration was found by the doctor who was called upon immediately after the accident. Artificial respiration and external cardiac massage were started and patient was sent to our hospital for further resuscitation. He arrived in our emergency clinic at 9: 00 a.m. but no heart beat, nor respiration could be detected. Resuscitation with oxygen, intracardiac injections with adrenalin and isoprel all failed after 40 minutes continuous resuscitation attempts.

Past history given by other members of his delegation revealed "heart disease" and "arrhythmia".

Diagnosis: Sudden death of cardiac origin.

His wife was present during the resuscitation attempts. The body was embalmed on the same day as requested by the embassy.

2. 尸体解剖证明（Certificate of autopsy）

尸体解剖证明

×××先生，35岁，谷玛水电站中国技术组技术员，2017年9月7日进行爆炸时头部被一沉重木头击中，2017年9月10日在罗蒂分克医院逝世。

2017年9月7日，患者在潘谷玛医院治疗，而后于同一天在塞格巴韦尼克松纪念医院治疗，进行了包括手术在内的一切治疗和处理。

为进一步加强手术治疗，患者被转移至罗蒂分克医院，在此最终死亡，为主治医生、中国专家杨先生所证实。

尸体立即转至弗里敦康纳特医院进行死后检查。

2017年9月12日在康纳特医院对尸体进行死后检查和解剖，尸体由卢先生——谷玛水电站组长辨认无误。

死后检查发现：尸体具有中年人尸体的特点，眼结合膜苍白，头发剃光。

右侧顶骨区有一10cm×20cm大小的头皮撕裂伤，该撕裂伤用黑丝线缝合，共9针。

打开头皮时，其整个内表面及右侧颞骨顶骨整个外表面可见广泛血肿，右侧顶骨亦有凹陷性骨折。

开颅时，硬脑膜下有出血及大量血肿，血流至硬脑膜下腔。

右侧顶骨区亦有脑压缩、脑表面出血及散在性瘀斑。

脑组织肿胀、松软、苍白。

双肺有斑点样实变。

心脏软、松、空。

胃肠扩张，有空气及液体。

肝、脾、肾十分苍白，此外均正常。

膀胱及生殖器正常。

死后尸体解剖发现要点

右侧顶骨头皮撕裂伤

右侧顶骨凹陷性骨折

硬膜下血肿

脑内血肿

脑水肿

支气管肺炎

血容量减少性休克

死　　因

主要死因：急性硬膜下及脑内血肿

先行死因：脑水肿及支气管肺炎

立即死因：血容量减少性休克

病理医生：×××

日期：2017 年 9 月 13 日

Certificate of Autopsy

Mr. ×××, thirty-five, a technician of the Guma Hydroelectric

Project, Chinese Technical Team, died on September 10, 2017, at Rotijunk Hospital after he had been struck on the head by a heavy log on September 7, 2017, while blasting.

He was first seen at Panguma Hospital and later at Nixon Memorial Hospital in Segbwema on the same day—September 7, 2017, and all possible medical management and treatment including surgery were done.

For further postoperative management, the patient was transferred to Rotijunk Hospital where he finally died. This was certified by the medical doctor in charge—Mr. Yang, a Chinese expert.

The body was immediately referred to Connaught Hospital in Freetown for post mortem examination.

A complete post mortem examination and section were done on the body on September 12, 2017, at Connaught Hospital Mortuary. The body was identified by Mr. Lu, the Director of the Guma Hydroelectric Project.

Post Mortem Findings—the body was that of a young man with pale conjunctiva. Hair on the head was completely shaved.

There was a scalp laceration of 10cm × 20cm in the right parietal region that had been sutured with black silk having a total number of nine stitches.

When opened the scalp, there was an extensive haematoma all over the internal surface of the scalp and the external surface of right temporo-parietal bone. There was also a depressed fracture of the right parietal bone.

When I opened the skull, I found haemorrhage and massive haematoma under the dura mater with bleeding into the subdural space.

There was also compression of the brain in the right parietal region with bleeding over the surface of the brain and scattered petechial haemorrhage.

The brain tissue was fairly swollen, soft and pale.

Lungs—patchy consolidation in both lungs.

Heart—soft, flabby, empty.

Stomach and intestines were distended with air and fluid.

Liver, spleen, kidneys fairly pale but normal otherwise.

Urinary bladder and genitalia were normal.

Post Mortem Summary

Right parietal scalp laceration.

Depressed fracture of right parietal bone.

Subdural haematoma.

Intracerebral haemotoma.

Cerebral edema.

Bronchopneumonia.

Hypovolemic shock.

Cause of Death

Primary: Acute subdural and intracerebral haematoma.

Antecedent: Cerebral edema and bronchopneumonia.

Immediate: Hypovolemic shock.

MEDICAL OFFICER: Dr. …

DATE: 13/9/2017

3. 出院证明（Discharge summary）

出 院 证 明

姓名：×××　　性别：女　　年龄：28 岁

病历号：32141　　入院日期：2017 年 4 月 6 日

出院日期：2017 年 4 月 21 日

诊断：慢性化脓性中耳炎（右耳）

病史及住院经过：

右耳反复流出臭味脓液 15 天、右乳突有压痛。检查发现右外耳道有脓液流出，鼓膜穿孔，X 线片显示鼓膜右乳突有骨质破坏，诊断为慢性化脓性中耳炎。

于 2017 年 4 月 11 日进行了右乳突根治术及鼓膜成形术，手术顺利，术后恢复良好。

出院医嘱：

（1）充足的营养、休息和睡眠，避免受凉；

（2）休息 10 天；

（3）切忌使劲擤鼻子；

（4）20 天后来我院门诊复查。

Discharge Summary

Name: ×××　　Sex: female　　Age: 28　　Case No.: 32141

Date of Admission (DOA): April 6, 2017

Date of Discharge (DOD): April 21, 2017

Diagnosis: chronic suppurative otitis media (right)

Simple history and course in hospital:

She was hospitalized with recurrent foul smelling pus from her right ear for 15 days. Examinations of the ears showed there was some purulent discharge in her right external canal with perforation of the tympanic membrane and tenderness over the right mastoid. X–ray film showed a bony destruction in the right mastoid. She was diagnosed as suffering from chronic suppurative otitis media.

Radical operation of the right and tympanoplastic operation were done on April 11, 2017. The course of the operation was good. She recovered well after the operation.

Discharge orders:

(1) Get adequate nourishment, rest and sleep, and avoid catching colds;

(2) Rest for 10 days;

(3) Be sure not to blow nose too violently;

(4) Come to the out-patient department for check-up in 20 days.

第八节   处方常用拉丁文缩写
（Common used Latin-abbreviations in prescription）

a., AA, aa	ana	各,每个,各同量
A. Add.	adde	加入
a.c.	ante cibum	饭前（服用）
ad	ad	至,加至
Ad us. ext.	ad usum externum	供外用
ad us. int	ad usum internum	供内用
Agit.	agita, agitetur	振荡,搅拌,摇动
a. j.	ante jentaculum	早饭前
a. m. , A.M.	ante meridiem	午前,上午
amp.	ampulla	安瓿（剂）,针剂
a. p.	ante prandium	午饭前
aq.	aqua	水
aq. ad.	aquam ad ….	加水至……
aq. dest.	aqua destillata	蒸馏水
a. u. agit	ante usum agitetur	用时摇匀
b. i. d.	bis in die	每日 2 次
B. P.	Britannica pharmacopceia	英国药典（标准）
c.	cum	和,用,与,以
C.	centigradus	摄氏温度表计

Cant.	cante	注意
caps., cap.	capsulae, capsula	胶囊（剂）
caps. gel.	capsulae gelatinosae	明胶胶囊（剂）
c. c.	centimeter cubicu	毫升，1mm^3
c. m.	cras mane	明日早晨
co., comp.	compositus	复方的，复合的
col.	collutorium	漱口剂
collun.	collunarium	洗鼻剂
collyr.	collyrum	洗眼剂
conc.	concentratus	浓缩的
crem.	cremor	乳剂
cryst.	crystallisatus, crystallus	已结晶的，结晶
D.	da, datur, detur	给予，应给予
d.	dosis	一次（用）量
de. , dec.	decoctum	炼剂，煎剂
Dil.	Dilue	稀释之
dil.	dilutus	稀释过的
Div.	Divide	分成（几份）
div. in p. aeq.	divide in partes aequales	分成等量
Div. in pulv.	Divide in pulveres	分成散剂
N. 6	numero sex	分成6包
D. S. , d. s.	Da, signa	给予（并）标明（用途）
D. t. d.	Da (dentur) tales doses	给予（数个同量）
Dt. d. No XⅡ	Da tales doses numero 12	给予同量12个
e. g.	exempi gratia	例如
em., emul.	emulsio	乳剂
ess.	essentia	香精
ext. extr	extractum	浸膏
F. Ft., ft.	Fiat, fiant	制作，制成

Fac	Facio	制成
fl.	fluidus	液体（的）
fort.	fortis	强的，浓的
g.	gramma	克
garg.	gargarisma	漱口水
Gr., gr.	granum	格令
gtt., gutt.	gutta, guttae	滴
h.	hora	小时
h. n.	hac nocte	今晚
h. n.s.	hac nocte sumendum	今晚服用
h. s.	hora somni	临睡前
i. a.	injectio arteriosa	动脉注射
i. c.	injectio (cavernae) cordis	心腔注射
i. d.	injectio dermica	皮内注射
i. e.	id est	即
i. h.	injectio hypodermica	皮下注射
i. m.	injectio muscularis	肌肉注射
i. p.	injectio abdominalis	腹腔注射
i. t.	injectio thecae (vaginae)	鞘内注射
i. v.	injectio venosa	静脉注射
i. v.gtt.	in venas guttatim	静脉滴注
inf.	infusum	浸剂
inhal.	inhalatio	吸入剂
inj.	injectio	注射（剂）
kg.	kilogramma	千克
lb	libra	磅
lin.	linimentum	擦剂
liq.	liquor	液剂
lot.	lotio	洗剂
M., m.	misce, misceatur	混合，使混合

m. d.	modo dicto	用法面授
m. d. a.	more dicto applicandum	依照指示的方法应用
M.D.S.	misce, da, signa; misceatur detur, signetur	混合,给予,标明用法
m. f. m.	misce, fiat mixtura	混合制成合剂
m. f. p.	misce, fiat pulvis	混合制成粉剂
mg.	milligramma	毫克
mist.	mistura	合剂
mixt.	mixtura	合剂
ml.	millilitra	毫升
moll.	mollis	软的
m. t. XII	mitte tales numero 12	给予同量12个
O. D.	oculus dexter	右眼
ol.	oleum	油
O. L. (S.)	oculus laevus (sinister)	左眼
oz. (unc.)	ounce (uncia)	盎司
O. U.	oculi utri	两眼
past.	pasta	糊剂
p. c.	post cibum	饭后
p. c.%	per centum	百分之
pig.	pigmentum	涂剂
pil.	pilula, pilulae	丸剂
p. m.	post meridiem	午后
p. o.	per os	口服,内服
ppt.	praecipitatum	调制的
p. r. n.	pro re nata	必要时（用）
pro n.	pro narcosi	麻醉用
pulv.	pulvis	粉剂
q. d.	quaque die	每日（一次）

q. 6h.	quaque 6 hora	每 6 小时一次
q. i. d.	quater in die	每日 4 次
q. o. d.	quaque omni die	每隔日一次
q. h.	quaque hora	每小时一次
q. s.	quantum sufficit, quantum satis	适量
Rp, Rx	recipe	取
S., Sig	sign	标记, 注明（服用或应用方法）
Sir., Syr.	sirupus, syrupus	糖浆
Sol.	solutus, solutio	溶液
S.O.S.	si opus sit	需要时用之
Ss., ss	semisse	（用）半（量）
St., stat.	Statim	立即（用）急!
Soppos.	suppositorium	栓剂
Syr.	syrupus	糖浆
tab.	tabella	片剂
t. i. d.	ter in die	一日三次
tinct. , tr.	tinctura	酊剂
troch.	trochioscus	锭剂
ung. , ungt.	unguentum	软膏
us. ext.	usus externus	外用
us. int.	usus internus	内服

第九节   合同与协议
(Contract and agreement)

合同和协议书是双方或几方对某事或某问题取得一致意见并确定了各自的权利和义务后达成的条文。合同和协议书使这些意见和权利义务都用书面形式固定下来,以利双方执行并作为书面凭证。遇到纠纷,可以此为证,辨明是非曲直,并督促当事人履行其所承诺的义务。协议书和合同一般包括以下几个部分:名称、正文、签署日期、地点、签字。下面列出几种合同、协议书供参考。

1. 聘约合同(Contract of employment)

聘 约 合 同

××医学院药理教研室(聘方)聘请×××博士(受聘方)为药理教师。双方本着友好合作的精神,同意签订并遵守下列条件:

(1)聘期为一年,自 2016 年 9 月 1 日起至 2017 年 8 月 31 日止。

(2)受聘方的工作任务,经双方确定如下:

①担任药理教研室师资和进修生的培训工作;

②从事药理学课程教学工作,指导学生和教师开展药理学术活动;

③编写药理学教材和补充读物以及进行其他与药理学有关的工作;

④每周工作量为 18~20 课时;

⑤受聘方每周工作 5 天,每天 8 小时。受聘方按照中国政府规定的节、假日放假,按照学校规定的寒暑假休假。

(3)聘方每月支付给受聘方工资人民币 5 000 元,并为受聘方提供各种应享受的待遇。

(4)受聘方入境、离境和过境时必须遵守中国政府有关外国人居住、工资福利及旅行的一系列管理规定,并遵守聘方的工作制度。

(5)聘方欢迎受聘方在工作中提出意见,并在条件允许时予以采纳。受聘方遵守聘方决定,积极工作,完成工作任务。

（6）双方均不得无故解除合同。聘方如果要求中途结束合同，除按照待遇条件承担受聘方的有关费用外，须给受聘方增发一个月的工资作为补偿金并于一个月以内安排受聘方及其家属回国。如果受聘方中途提出辞职，聘方自同意之日起即停发工资，受聘方不再享受各种待遇条件。受聘方及其家属回国的一切费用均由本人自理。

（7）本合同自受聘方到职之日起生效，聘期届满，即自行失效。如一方要求延长聘期，必须在合同期满前向对方提出，经双方协商确认后，可另行签定延长聘期合同。

（8）本合同在执行中如有争议，由双方协商解决。

（9）本合同用中文和英文两种文字写成。两种文本具有同等效力。

聘　　方　　　　　受　聘　方

CONTRACT OF EMPLOYMENT

The Pharmacology. Department of...Medical College (the engaging party) has engaged Dr. ... (the engaged party) as a teacher of pharmacology. The two parties, in the spirit of friendship and cooperation, have agreed to sign and comply with the below stated conditions.

(1) The term of service is one year, from September 1, 2016 to August 31, 2017.

(2) The duties of the engaged party is mutually agreed to be:

a) Training teachers of pharmacology and students taking refresher courses.

b) Conducting pharmacology classes and advising students and teachers on pharmacological activities.

c) Compiling pharmacology textbooks and supplementary teaching material, undertaking other work connected with the pharmacology.

d) Having 18 up to 20 teaching periods in a week.

e) The engaged party works five days a week and eight hours a day. The engaged party will have legal holidays as prescribed by the Chinese Government. The vacation is fixed by the school calendar.

(3) The engaging party agrees to pay the engaged party a monthly salary of five thousand yuan (Chinese currency) and provide him with various benefits.

(4) The engaged party must observe the regulations of the Chinese Government concerning residence, wages and benefits, and travel for foreigners when entering, leaving and passing through the PRC territories, and must follow the work schedules of the engaging party.

(5) The engaging party will welcome any suggestion put forward by the engaged party and will render favourable consideration when circumstances permit. The engaged party will abide by the decisions of the engaging party and work in the spirit of active cooperation to accomplish assigned tasks.

(6) Neither party shall, without sufficient cause or reason, cancel the contract.

If the engaging party finds it imperative to terminate the contract, then, in addition to bearing the corresponding expenses for wages and benefits, it must pay the engaged party one month's extra salary as compensation allowance, and arrange for him and his family's return to their own country within a mouth.

If the engaged party submit his (her) resignation within the contract period, the engaging party will be relieved of the responsibility for wages and benefits as of the date the engaged's resignation is accepted and approved by the engaging party. In addition, the engaged party must provide for his and his family's return to the country of origin without expense to the engaging institution.

(7) The present contract becomes effective on the first day of service herein stipulated and ceases to be effective on the last of service. If either party wishes to renew the contract, negotiations must be entered prior to the expiration of the original contract. Upon agreement by both parties through consultation a new contract may be signed.

(8) Should any matter, not provided for in this contract, arise during the course of performance, it will be settled through consultation by the two parties.

(9) The Chinese translation of this contract will faithfully represent the spirit of the English version and shall be binding on both parties.

————————————   ————————————
　(the engaging party)   　(the engaged party)

2. 延长聘期合同（Extension of employment contract）

延长聘期合同

×× 医学院药理教研室（聘方）与 ××× 博士（受聘方）根据共同的愿望，商定延长聘期二年，自 2016 年 9 月 1 日起 2018 年 8 月 31 日止。双方确认，2015 年 7 月 12 日签订的合同所提各项内容，在延长聘期内继续有效。

————————————   ————————————
　　聘　　方　　　　　　　　受　聘　方

EXTENSION OF EMPLOYMENT CONTRACT

The Pharmacology Department of... Medical College (the engaging party) and Dr. ... (the engaged party), motivated by their common desire, agree to extend the employment contract for two years, from September 1, 2016 to August 31, 2018. The two parties affirm that all stipulations contained in the original employment contract signed on July 12, 2015 remain in effect throughout the extension.

_____   _____
(The Engaging Party)   (The Engaged Party)

3. 建立学术交流计划的协议书（Agreement on establishment of an exchange program）

建立学术交流计划的协议书

为建立在美国训练年轻教师和在中国帮助教学的交流计划，中国承德医学院和美国路易斯维尔大学经友好协商，达成本协议。

（1）目的和目标：

双方认为，通过建立学术交流计划，能促进承德医学院和路易斯维尔大学之间的学术交流、相互了解和友谊，进而在双方互利的基础上，加强友好合作和联系。

（2）路易斯维尔大学的职责：

路易斯维尔大学每年提供二名奖学金名额，来培养从承德医学院基础教研室挑选出的年轻教师。这二名年轻教师在美国的生活费由路易斯维尔大学负担，从中国至路易斯维尔市的旅费由承德医学院负担。

（3）承德医学院的职责：

①承德医学院每年从路易斯维尔大学邀请一名教授或副教

授来承德帮助八年制班讲授医学课程,时间为 3~4 个月。他或她在承德停留期间,承德医学院每月提供食宿和生活费（大约 4 000 元人民币）。但承德医学院不负担其从美国至中国的往返国际旅费。

②承德医学院荣幸地聘请路易斯维尔大学 ×× 教授作为此协议的联络员。××× 教授愿意为以上有关①和②项的工作无偿地做联络工作。

中华人民共和国　　美利坚合众国
承德医学院代表　　路易斯维尔大学代表

AGREEMENT ON ESTABLISHMENT OF AN EXCHANGE PROGRAM

This agreement has been reached by friendly consultation between Chengde Medical College (CMC), China and University of Louisville (UL), U.S.A. to establish an exchange program for training the junior faculty members in the United States and helping the teaching in China.

(1) AIMS AND PURPOSES:

Both sides acknowledge that by setting up the exchange program, it would promote the academic exchange, understanding and friendship between Chengde Medical College and University of Louisville, thus enhancing friendly co−operation and contracts on the basis of mutual benefit.

(2) OBLIGATION OF UL:

University of Louisville will offer two fellowships annually to train two junior faculty members of CMC who have been selected among the preclinical departments. The annual stipend will be paid by UL and the travel expenses covered from China to Louisville, KY, U.S.A. will be paid by CMC.

(3) OBLIGATION OF CMC:

①Chengde Medical College would like to invite one Professor or associate professor of UL to spend 3 or 4 months in Chengde to help the teaching of eight-year medical program. While he or she is in Chengde, CMC will supply the accommodation and a living allowance (approximately ￥4 000 per month). But CMC won't pay his or her travel expenses from U.S.A. to China.

②CMC would be pleased to have Professor … of the University of Louisville as its liaison at gratis for our future communication concerned Item ①to②.

Chengde Medical College, the people's Republic of China	University of Louisville United States of America

4. 建立研究生班的协议书（Agreement on establishment of graduate class）

中华人民共和国承德医学院与美利坚合众国杜布克大学关于举办护理学硕士研究生班协议书

为了进一步加强中美两国的学术和文化交流，经两校充分协商，双方达成协议如下：

（1）杜布克大学同意与承德医学院合作，在承德医学院举办护理学硕士研究生班。

（2）杜布克大学护理学硕士研究生学位课为十门，三十学分。根据中国的实际情况将增设两门课，因此，杜布克大学在承德医学院举办的护理学硕士研究生班为十二门课，三十六学分,每年安排六门课程,二年内完成,结束时举行综合考试。

下列课程仅作参考:

①护理理论的发展

②护理科研

③护理行政管理

④护理教育

⑤健康与疾病的心理社会适应

⑥护理程序与责任制护理

⑦老年和慢性病护理

⑧急症护理

⑨临终护理

⑩家庭健康护理

⑪选修课两门

（3）参加护理学硕士研究生班的学生进入 MSN 学习前必须具有学士学位资格证书,TOFEL 成绩在 500 分以上或有 EPT 考试合格成绩。

（4）杜布克大学将为该班选派有博士（或硕士）学位的专职教授来担任此班十二门课的讲授任务。杜布克大学选派的兼职教授,必须经承德医学院院长批准后,方可任教。

（5）杜布克大学在开课前四个月将有关教材,包括教学大纲和教科书寄到承德医学院。

（6）护理学硕士研究生班每门课授课时间至少持续3~4周。负责实习的医院应由美国衣阿华中央护理委员会批准。

（7）杜布克大学的教授在承德医学院授课期间的食宿由承德医学院按照外籍教授标准提供。如这些教授选择在外食宿承德医学院则不负担其费用。如教授携配偶或子女来华,其费用自理。如家属在校内用餐,每人每天交纳三美元。家属如与教授同住一室,不另收费。承德医学院不负责教授家属的旅游费用。

（8）杜布克大学来执教的教授的工资及国际旅费由该大学

负责。应承德医学院邀请任教的二名中国教授的工资同杜布克大学任教的教授工资相等。

（9）学费为每个学生每学分146美元，按教学计划规定的30个学分计算，每个学生学费总数为4 380美元。

（10）此班学生人数为25~30人。承德医学院为杜布克大学提供学费共109 500美元。如有剩余由承德医学院支配。

（11）根据中国卫生部对外国专家医疗待遇的有关规定，承德医学院负责杜布克大学教授在承授课期间的医疗费。但规定之外的医疗费用由教授个人负担（如镶牙、整容等）。在中国工作期间的其他保险问题由教授自理。

（12）杜布克大学的教授因工作需要的所有交通、通讯费用由承德医学院提供，工作之外的交通、通讯费用则由教授本人负担。

（13）此班结束时，由杜布克大学授以护理学硕士学位，此学位与杜布克大学在美国所授学位相同，并得到美国中北区高等教育评审委员会的认可。

（14）协议书草案将于2016年3月在承德医学院签署。护理学硕士研究生班将于2016年9月1日开始。

（15）学生来自河北省和全国其他各省，从港澳地区最大限度选择十名。

（16）此协议中英文正本二份，副本二份，具有同等效力。经中国××市政府和美国中北区高等教育评审委员会批准后，自双方校长在杜布克大学签字之日起开始生效。

———————————————　　　　———————————————

承德医学院院长（签字）　　　杜布克大学校长（签字）

日期：　　　　　　　　　　　日期：

THE AGREEMENT ON ESTABLISHMENT OF M.S.N. GRADUATE CLASS BETWEEN THE CHENGDE MEDICAL COLLEGE (CMC), P.R.C. AND THE UNIVERSITY OF DUPUQUE (UD), U.S.A.

In order to further strengthen the academic and culture exchange between China and United States, the two sides have reached the following agreement after a thorough discussion of these two universities.

(1) The UD approves a co-operation with CMC to run a MASTER OF SCIENCE IN NURSING (MSN) program in CMC.

(2) The MSN degree offered by the UD includes ten subjects and 30 credits hours. Two more subjects are being added in accordance with practical conditions in China. Therefore, the MSN graduate class run by the UD will have 12 subjects and 36 credits hours which will be operated at the CMC. Six subjects have to be finished in each year and all 12 subjects will be completed within two years and then a comprehensive exam will be given. We suggest the following subjects for reference only:

①The development of nursing theory.

②Nursing research.

③Nursing administration.

④Nursing Education.

⑤Psycho-social adaptation of health and diseases.

⑥Nursing process and primary nursing.

⑦Nursing of the elderly & chronic diseases.

⑧Nursing of acute diseases.

⑨Nursing care of the dying patient.

⑩Family health nursing.

⑪Two elective courses.

(3) Students who apply into the MSN program must possess the qualified certificate of B.S. degree and above 500 marks of TOFEL or the result of EPT (English Proficiency Test) before they are admitted.

(4) The UD will select teachers from their full–time Professors with Ph. D. or M.S. degree to hold responsibility in lecturing of these 12 subjects in China. The concurrent (part–time) Professors selected by the UD can only hold the teaching post after the approval of the President of CMC.

(5) The UD should send the related teaching materials, including teaching programs and textbooks to CMC preferably 4 months ahead of the beginning of teaching.

(6) In this MSN program the lecture hours of each subject will last at least 3–4 weeks. The hospitals attached to the training should be approved by Iowa Central Nursing Committees of America.

(7) The CMC will bear the expenses of board and lodging for the Professors come from the UD during their stay in CMC according to the standard for foreign Professors. CMC will not cover expenses of board and lodging of the Professors who prefer to stay outside of the College. The expenses of their accompanied spouse and children will be borne by the Professors themselves. Three meals per day is charged for U.S. $ 3.0 per person if their family members are chosen to stay with the professors on the College campus. The dependents won't be charged for lodging fee if they stay in the same room with the professors. CMC will not be responsible for the traveling expenses of their dependents.

(8) The UD will bear the salary and international traveling expenses for their professors while they come to Chengde performing

their teaching duty. The salary of two Chinese professors invited by CMC will be given according to the standard of professors from the UD.

(9) Student will be charged the tuition fee for U.S. $146 per credit hour. The total amount of tuition for whole course will be U.S. $4 380, based on the calculation of total 30 credit hours.

(10) 25 to 30 students will be enrolled in the class. CMC will reimburse the UD with a total amount of U.S.A. 109,500 for the tuition. If it shows a small surplus, CMC will make its own allocation.

(11) CMC will be responsible to pay the expenses of medical treatment of Professors during their stay in Chengde according to the regulation of the Ministry of Health of China and to the medical treatment for foreign experts. Any expense outside of the regulation will be covered by the Professors themselves, such as artificial tooth inserting and face-lifting, etc. Furthermore, other insurances will also be covered by the Professors themselves.

(12) CMC will provide the Professors of the UD with expenses for any business communication if it is required by their work. However, CMC won't pay the expenses for their private business.

(13) When the class is complete, the UD will confer the degree of MSN to each student. The degree certificate is the same as the one awarded by the UD in the States and approved by the Northern Central Higher Educational Evaluation Committee in U.S.A.

(14) The draft of the agreement will be signed in March, 2016 at CMC. The MSN graduate class will begin at September 1 , 2016.

(15) The students come from Hebei region and all parts of China. Maximum ten students will be selected from the region of Hongkong and Macao.

(16) Two texts in English and Chinese, two copies each, are equally authentic. After approval by Chengde Municipal Government

in China and the Northern Central Higher Educational Evaluation Committee, in U.S.A. the draft of agreement will go into effect from he date of signature by the two sides in the UD.

(Signature)　　　　　　　　(Signature)
Chengde Medical College　　The University of Dupuque

第十节　论文摘要
（Abstract of dissertation）

论文摘要是对论文或文献所做的扼要摘述，它以精练的字句向读者介绍论文的主要内容。文摘一般包括目的、材料和方法、结果和结论四个部分。字数为 200 字左右。前有标题及作者姓名、地址，后有关键词（key words）。

文摘的标题是对论文的高度概括，它一般是名词性短语。文摘的目的表明了研究工作的主旨。材料和方法部分则介绍了研究工作中所用到的材料和方法。结果部分包括观察和实验所获得的客观事实和数据。结论部分则是作者说明本研究工作所获得结果的理论和实践意义，提出自己的观点。

文摘的目的、材料和方法、结果这三部分通常采用过去时态，而结论部分则采用现在时态、现在完成时态或将来时态。

英语文摘的格式随刊物不同而略有不同，故撰写时应参照拟投稿的刊物的文摘格式。

1. 儿童重症肌无力的手术疗效

儿童重症肌无力的手术疗效

［摘要］**目的**：分析儿童重症肌无力的手术疗效。**方法**：2011—2014 年，共有 36 例儿童重症肌无力患者行胸腺切除术，

年龄4~14岁,病程2个月~8年,按 Osserman 分型,其中 I 型 27例, II a 型6例, II b 型2例, III 型1例,疗效评价分治愈和改善。**结果**:本组治愈者占13.9%,改善69.4%,有效率(治愈或改善)达83.3%,无恶化或住院死亡者。**结论**:疗效与病程长短、具体分型及病理类型有关,与性别年龄无关,随访结果令人满意。

　　关键词:重症肌无力;胸腺切除

Effects of Thymectomy on Myasthemia Gravis in Children

[Abstract] Objective: To analyze the surgical effects of thymectomy on Myasthenia Gravis (MG) in children. **Methods:** Totally 36 children with MG were treated by thymectomy from 2011 to 2014.Their ages ranged from 4 to 14 years old, and symptom duration from 2 months to 8 years. According to Osserman classification, Type I was observed in 27 cases, Type II a in 6 cases, Type II b in 2 cases and Type III in 1 case. The relevant evaluation of effects falls into two types: the cured ones and improved ones. **Results:** Patients who were cured accounts for 13.9% and those who got improved for 69.4%. The rate of efficiency (including both cases) amounts to 83.3%, and no patient suffered exacerbated condition or died. **Conclusions:** The medical treatment turns out to be related with the duration of the disease, pathological types and clinical classification but irrelevant to sex and age. The results obtained from follow-up visits are satisfactory.

　　Key words: Myasthenia gravis; Thymectomy

2. 沙棘籽油治疗酒精性肝硬化的报告

沙棘籽油治疗酒精性肝硬化的报告摘要

酒精性肝硬化目前尚无特效疗法。我科于 2010 年 6 月收治 1 例酒精性肝硬化患者，应用沙棘籽油治疗，收到较好效果。现报告如下。

病历摘要：患者，男，58 岁。主诉"上腹胀痛 20 天"入院。既往有近 20 年饮白酒史，每日 300~500ml，否认传染性肝炎史。查体：面色黝黑，皮肤、巩膜轻度黄染，肝质中，无压痛。肝功能、B 超 CT 等检查均符合肝硬化改变。同位素放射免疫肝功能检查，透明质酸梅 >640μg/L，铁蛋白 >500μg/L，肝胆酸 52.36μmol/L。乙肝系列等病毒标志物检查均呈阴性。

诊断和治疗结果：单纯服用沙棘油，每日 3 次，每次 10ml，连服 70d，复查肝功能及同位素放射免疫肝功能等项目均正常，其中，透明质酸酶 <160μg/L，铁蛋白 <240μg/L，甘胆酸 <8.94μg/L。

讨论：本例患者应用沙棘油使肝功能和同位素肝功能等检查恢复正常，这可能与该药提高机体免疫功能、增强抗病能力、改善病灶微循环、促进组织细胞再生有关。

Seabuck Seed Oil for Alcoholic Hepatocirrhosis: A Case Report

There hasn't been a specific drug for alcoholic hepatocirrhosis at present. We reported a case admitted in June, 2010 for alcoholic hepatocirrhosis treated with seabuck seed oil with satisfactory result.

Case History

A patient aged 58 reported a 20–day history of epigastric distention complicated with hypodynamia. The patient had a 20–year history of alcoholic drinking, with 300–500ml daily, but denied the history of infectious hepatitis. Physical examinations showed a dark complexion, slight xanthochromia of the skin and sclea. Liver was found to be moderate and no tenderness was found. Examinations of liver function, Bultrasound and CT scanning all suggested hepatocirrhosis. Isotope radioimmunoassy of hepatofunction showed hyaluronate>640μg/L, ferritin>500μg/L, hepatic acid 52.36μmol/L. Serial hepatitis B virus–marking tests were negative.

Diagnosis and Results of Treatment

The patients was given seabuck seed oil, 10ml each time and 3 times daily, and consecutively for 70 days. Tests for evaluation of hepatic function and isotope radioimmunoassy showed normal: hyaluronate <160μg/L, ferritin <240μg/L, hepatic acid <8.94μg/L.

Discussion

In this case, seabuck seed oil was applied with the result that the tests of hepatic function and isotope radioimmunoassy became normal. This might be related to the strengthening of the immunity of body, thus increasing resistance to the disease, the improvement of micro–circulation of the focus, and the enhancement of the formation of tissue cells through the use of seabuck seed oil.

3. 妇女生育健康：早年、成年期体质量指数的影响

妇女生育健康：早年、成年期
体质量指数的影响

背景：体重过轻和过重的妇女发生月经问题和不育症的概率较高，但目前证据不尽一致，尤其是关于肥胖发生的年龄对上述问题的影响方面意见不同。**目的**：确定成年期和儿童期的体质量指数（BMI）对妇女生育健康的影响。**方法**：根据2008

年英国出生人群研究所提供的 5 799 名女性身高，（7、11、16、23 和 33 岁时的）体重和生殖数据体质量指数以体重 / 身高 ^{2} 计算。根据不同年龄的分段来确定体重过重和肥胖。33 岁时报告的与生育有关的问题包括：月经问题（16 岁时也有同样报告），孕期高血压和低生育力。**结果**：初经期早与 16 岁前的月经问题有关，但是，这种关系到 33 岁不复存在。在调整其他干扰因素后，23 岁时发生的肥胖和 7 岁时发生的肥胖都与 33 岁前的月经问题有关。（OR 分别为 1.75 和 1.59）。在调整其他干扰因素后，23 岁时发生的肥胖导致孕期高血压的概率增加。（OR=2.73）。与这些发现一致的是，在调整其他干扰因素后，23 岁时发生肥胖的妇女在无任何避孕的情况下 12 月内不易受孕（RR=0.69）。**结论**：成年早期的体重过重和肥胖似乎较易导致月经问题、孕期高血压和低生育力。除了月经问题外，儿童期的体质量指数与妇女的生殖健康无多大关系。

Women's Reproductive Health: The Role of Body Mass Index in Early and Adult Life

Background: Higher risks of menstrual problems and infertility have been found in underweight and overweight women but evidence is inconsistent especially in relation to the effect of age of onset of obesity. **Objective:** To determine whether body mass index (BMI) in adulthood or childhood affects the reproductive health of women. **Methods:** Heights, weights (at 7, 11, 16, 23 and 33y) and reproductive data were available for 5 799 females in the 2008 British birth cohort study. Body mass index (BMI) was calculated as weight/height ^{2}. Age-specific cut-offs were used to define overweight and obesity. Reproductive outcomes reported at age 33 included: menstrual problems (also reported at 16 y), hypertension in pregnancy and subfertility. **Results:** Early menarcheal age was associated with higher risks of menstrual problems by 16 y but this relationship did not persist to 33y. Obesity at 23 y and obesity at 7 y both independently increased the risk of menstrual problems by age 33 (OR=1.75, OR=1.59 respectively) after adjusting for other confounding factors. Obesity at 23 y increased the risk of hypertension in pregnancy (OR=2.37), after adjusting for confounders. Consistent with these findings, obese women at 23 y were less likely to conceive within 12 months of unprotected intercourse after adjustment for confounders (RR=0.69). **Conclusions:** Overweight and obesity in early adulthood appears to increase the risk of menstrual problems, hypertension in pregnancy and subfertility. Other than menstrual problems, childhood body mass index had little impact on the reproductive health of women.

4. 木贼对大鼠心功能的影响

木贼对大鼠心功能的影响

[摘要]目的:研究木贼对心脏功能的影响。方法:建立新式离体作功心脏模型。用上海产 SJ-42 型四道生理记录仪测定生理参数左室收缩压（LVSP）、左室内压上升速率最大值（dP/dt$_{max}$）、左室舒张期末压（LVEDP）、左室内压下降速率最大值（-dP/dt$_{max}$）、冠脉流量（CF）、心率（HR）和心电图（ECG）。结果:经过适当剂量木贼药液灌注后的离体作功心脏与用药前自身对照比较,LVSP、dP/dt$_{max}$、-dP/dt$_{max}$、CF 增大,而 HR 变慢。结论:木贼有增强心脏收缩与舒张功能,有增加冠脉流量和减慢心率的作用。

[关键词]木贼;大鼠离体作功心脏;收缩与舒张功能;冠脉流量;心率

EFFECT OF EQUISETUM HIEMALE L ON THE PHYSIOLOGICAL CARDIAC PERFORMANCES OF RAT

[Abstract] Objective: To study the effect of Equisetum hiemale L on the cardiac performances. Methods: A new isolated working heart model was established. The physiological parameters of isolated working heart were recorded with a 4–channel polygraph system, model SJ–42, manufactured in Shang–hai, China. The present experiment describes the effect of Equisetum hiemale L on the left ventricular systolic pressure (LVSP), peak rate of LV pressure rise (dP/dt_{max}), left ventricular end–diastolic pressure (LVEDP), peak rate of LV pressure decline ($-dP/dt_{max}$), coronary flow (CF), heart rate (HR) and electrocardiogram (ECG). Results: The parameters LVSP, dP/dt_{max}, $-dP/dt_{max}$, and CF were higher and that the HR was slower after Equisetum hiemale L treatment when compared with the control. Conclusion: These finding suggest that the systole–diastolic performances became stronger and coronary flow increase and that the heart rate became slower after Equisetum hiemale L treatment.

[Key Words] Equisetum hiemale L; Rat isolated working heart; Systole–diastolic performances; Coronary flow; Heart rate.

5. 25例结核性腹膜炎误诊原因分析

25例结核性腹膜炎误诊原因分析

[摘要]本文分析了结核性腹膜炎误诊原因,认为综合医院的内科医生对现代结核性腹膜炎知识生疏,多不了解结核性腹膜炎的早期可疑症状,忽略了简便易行的腹部查体、腹部试穿及B超检查。因此,提高基层综合医院医师的诊断水平,注意综合细致地分析病人的症状、体征和化验结果是必要的。

[**关键词**]结核性腹膜炎；误诊

ANALYSIS OF MISDIAGNOSIS CAUSES IN 25 CASES OF TUBERCULOUS PERITONITIS

[**Abstract**] The misdiagnosis causes were analyzed in 25 patients with the tuberculous peritonitis. The authors found that the physicians working in a general hospital were not quite familiar with the modern knowledge of the early tuberculous peritonitis, most of them did not know the early suspicious symptoms of the disease, therefore they ignored the simple and convenient abdominal examination, experimental abdominocentesis and B–ultrasonic scanning. The results reveal that it is vital for the physicians serving in the local general hospital to raise the level of making correct diagnosis and the ability for analyzing symptoms, physical signs and the result of the laboratory examination.

[**Key Words**] Tuberculous peritonitis; Misdiagnosis

6. 胸腔镜术在内科的应用价值

胸腔镜术在内科的应用价值

[**摘要**]**目的**：探索内科医师掌握胸腔镜术对胸膜疾病诊断与治疗的实用性及可行性。**方法**：用纤维支气管及硬质胸腔镜对 345 例胸膜病在局麻下行开放式胸腔镜术，观察患者对手术的耐受性及安全性。**结果**：（1）病因诊断率：胸腔积液 245 例确定病因 227 例（92.7%），气胸 92 例确定病因 69 例（75.0%），胸膜肿块 8 例，均获得组织学诊断。（2）疗效：恶性胸腔积液 102 例，近期胸腔积液消失 80 例（78.4%），92 例气胸治愈 75 例（81.5%），28 例脓胸治愈 26 例（92.9%）。（3）安全性：98 例术中监护心电图、血氧饱和度、血压、呼吸、脉搏均无重要临床意义

改变。345 例中 24 例（7.0%）术中出现窦性心动过速。**结论：**（1）胸腔镜能窥视整个胸膜腔，在直视下活检是疑难胸膜疾病病因诊断的最佳方法。（2）难治性胸腔积液、常规治疗失败或复发性气胸、不宜手术者行胸腔镜介入治疗是有效而实用的方法。（3）局麻下行胸腔镜术操作简单、安全。

　[**关键词**]胸腔镜术；胸腔积液；气胸

The Value of Medical Thoracoscopy

[**Abstract**] **Objective:** To study the practicality and feasibility for a physician to diagnose and treat pleural diseases through thoracoscopy. **Methods:** To perform open thoracoscopy on 345 patients with a fibrobronchoscope or a hard thoracoscope under local anesthesia and evaluate the safety and tolerance of patients during the operation. **Results:** (1) Determination of etiology: in 92.7% (227/245 cases) of pleural effusion cases, 75.0% (69/92) of pneumothorax cases, etiologic causes have been determined and 8 cases of pleural tumors were diagnosed. (2) Therapeutic effectiveness: the response rate of malignant pleural effusions was 78.4% (80/102 cases). (3) Safety: during operation the ECG, SaO_2, BP, R, P of 98 patients did not show important changes. In 345 patients. 7% (24/345) showed sinus tachycardia. **Conclusions:** (1) Through thoracoscopy, we can observe the whole pleural cavity and can take biopsy specimen under direct observation. It is a good method to get the etiological diagnosis in cause-underdetermined pleural diseases. (2) It is effective and practical to treat difficult pleural effusion, the obstinate pneumothorax, or one that is not suitable for thoracic surgery. (3) It is safe and simple to apply the thoracoscopy under local anesthesia.

　[**Key words**] Thoracoscopy; Pleural effusion; Pneumothorax

7. 降主动脉瘤的腔内移植物治疗

<h2 style="text-align:center">降主动脉瘤的腔内移植物治疗</h2>

[摘要]目的：探讨腔内移植物治疗降主动脉瘤的可行性。**方法**：12例降主动脉瘤接受了血管腔内技术治疗，包括5例真性动脉瘤、6例 Stanford B 型夹层动脉瘤及1例假性动脉瘤。12枚支架型血管在局部(n=2)或全身麻醉(n=10)下经一侧股动脉切开安装在病变部位。 **结果**：腔内技术成功率100%。无瘤体破裂、截瘫及肢体缺血等并发症。早期并发症：3例早期内漏血。5例真性动脉瘤，4例被完全旷置，1例内漏转化为持续性。6例 Stanford B 型夹层入口，4例一期封堵满意，2例少量内漏自愈。4例假腔内完全血栓形成，2例部分形成。**结论**：腔内移植物治疗降主动脉瘤是一种安全、可靠、实用的新方法。但其远期治疗效果有待继续观察，尤其是夹层动脉瘤的腔内治疗具有更多的不确定性。

[关键词]主动脉瘤；心血管外科手术方法；支架；

<h2 style="text-align:center">Endovascular Stent–grafting of Descending
Thoracic Aortic Lesions</h2>

[Abstract] Objective: To discuss the feasibility of endoluminal stent–grafting for descending thoracic aortic lesions. Methods: Endovascular technique was used in 12 patients with descending thoracic aortic aneurysms (5patients), Stanford B dissections (6), and pseudoaneurysm (1). 12 straight stent–grafts were inserted via a femoral arteriotomy under local (2 patients) or general (10) anesthesia. Results: The procedure was technically successful in all patients without aneurysm rupture, paraplegia, and organs or limbs ischemia. There were 3 early endoleaks. Follow–up showed that 4 of 5 aortic aneurysms were excluded completely and one endoleak was changed into persistent. Four entries of 6 patient with Stanford B dissection were excluded and 2 early endoleaks were sealed during one month after operation. Four false lumen were filled completely and 2 false lumen were filled partly be thrombosis. **Conclusion:** Descending thoracic aortic stent-grafting is a safe, highly successful and feasible alternative to conventional surgery. The long-term result remains unclear, especially that of the endovascular repair of Stanford B dissection.

[**Key words**] Aortic aneurysm; Cardiovascular surgical procedure; Stents;

8. 267 例主髂动脉闭塞的手术治疗经验

267 例主髂动脉闭塞的手术治疗经验

[摘要]目的: 探讨肾动脉开口水平以下腹主动脉闭塞及髂动脉闭塞的手术方式选择及治疗经验。**方法**: 回顾性分析 267 例主、髂动脉闭塞患者的临床资料。结果: 267 例患者全部行手术治疗。行腹主动脉–髂（股）动脉人工血管转流术 145 例, 髂动脉—股动脉人工血管转流术 40 例, 股动脉—股动脉人工血管转流术 45 例, 腋动脉–股动脉人工血管转流术 37 例。总有效率为 96.5%, 围手术期病死率为 3.5%。267 例中 178 例得到随访, 平均随访时间 5 年 9 个月, 人工血管通畅率为 82.0%。结论: 对于年老、体弱者, 特别是全身一般状况较差, 伴有冠状动脉性心脏病、高血压、脑动脉硬化、脑梗死等慢性疾病的患者, 应采用腋动脉–（双）髂股动脉人工血管转流术或股动脉–股动脉人工转流术。

[关键词]动脉闭塞性疾病; 主动脉, 腹; 髂动脉; 人工血管

Experience of Arterial Occlusive Diseases of Abdominal Aorta and iliac Artery

[Abstract] Objective: To study the surgical treatment of infrarenal aortic and iliac arterial occlusive disease. Method: Analyzed 267 patients with arterial occlusive diseases of the abdominal aorta and iliac artery retrospectively. Results: All the patients were treated by surgery including aortic–iliac bypass in 145 patients, iliac–femoral bypass in 40, femoro–femoral bypass in 45, and axillo–femoral bypass in 37.Their total effective rate and perioperative motality were 96.5% and 3.5%, respectively. Of the 267 patients, 178 were followed up. The patency rate of prosthesis was 82.0%. Conclusions: Extra–anatomical bypass is a procedure of choice for high–risk patients, especially for those chronic patients with coronary heart disease, hypertension, cerebral arterial atherosclerosis, and brain infarction.

[Key word] Arterial occlusive diseases; Aorta, abdominal; Iliac artery; Blood vessel prosthesis

9. 腹腔镜手术治疗肾上腺嗜铬细胞瘤

腹腔镜手术治疗肾上腺嗜铬细胞瘤

[摘要]目的:探讨腹腔镜手术治疗肾上腺嗜铬细胞瘤的临床价值。方法:采用腹腔镜手术治疗肾上腺嗜铬细胞瘤7例,其中5例采用经腹腔途径,2例采用腹膜后途径。结果:6例成功,1例因术中损伤胰腺出血改为开放手术。随访10~48个月,患者血压正常,肿瘤局部无复发。结论:对直径<6cm的肾上腺嗜铬细胞瘤,只要术前准备充分,腹腔镜手术安全有效,有望替代开放手术成为首选的治疗方法。

[关键词]腹腔镜术;肾上腺;嗜铬细胞瘤

Laparoscopic Surgery for Adrenal Pheochromocytoma

[Abstract] Objective: To evaluate the application of laparoscopic surgery for adrenal pheochromocytoma. Method: 7 cases of adrenal pheochromocytoma were treated with laparoscopic surgery. The laparoscopic procedures included 5 transperitoneal and 2 retroperitoneal approaches. Results: Success was achieved in 6 cases while in the other one the procedure was transferred to open surgery because of pancreas injury with bleeding. Postoperative follow up has been 10~48 months. In all the patients blood pressure returned to normal and no residual tumors were found after laparoscopic surgery. Conclusions: As long as preoperative preparation was adequate, laparoscopic surgery could be safe and feasible for tumors smaller than 6 cm.

[Key word] Peritoneoscopy; Adrenal glands; Pheochromocytoma

10. 影响糖尿病患者心血管危险因素集簇现象的因素

影响糖尿病患者心血管危险因素集簇现象的因素

[摘要]目的:分析影响糖尿病患者多种心血管危险因素集簇现象的因素。方法:调查654例糖尿病患者并发症情况。计算出胰岛素抵抗指数,按照并存心血管危险因素(高血压、全身性肥胖、中心性肥胖、高胆固醇血症、低HDL-胆固醇血症)数量,进行分析。结果:并有3种以上的心血管危险因素明显地高于随机的单一因素并存的计算预测值,餐后胰岛素水平和胰岛素面积随危险因素的增加而增加。采用有性别差异的全身性

肥胖和中心性肥胖的诊断标准，女性糖尿病患者有更多的心血管危险因素。如果采用男女性别相同的诊断标准，这种并存多种心血管危险因素的性别差异则消失。多数患者的这些危险因素未得到良好的控制。**结论**：糖尿病多种心血管危险因素集簇是常见的，可能与高胰岛素血症及性别有关。

[**关键词**]糖尿病；心血管疾病；高胰岛素血症；肥胖；高血压；性

The Elements Affecting the Clustering of cardiovascular Risk Factors in Diabetic Patients

[**Abstract**] **Objective:** To investigate the factors affecting the clustering of cardiovascular risk factors in Chinese patients with diabetes. **Methods:** Six hundred and fifty-four patients with diabetes were examined comprehensively for diabetes complications and cardiovascular risk factors in a metropolitan hospital. Insulin resistance and secretion were also evaluated by measurement of glucose and insulin levels before and 2h after a meal. Results were analyzed according to patient groups stratified by the number of cardiovascular risk factors coexisting with diabetes. **Results:** Clustering of three or more of these factors with diabetes occurred greater than that by random one factor alone and was associated with postprandial hyperinsulinemia. Patients with more risk factors were more prone to macrovascular events. Using the commonly adopted lower threshold for diagnosing obesity and central obesity in women, there were more females with multiple risk factors. But the difference disappeared if the same criteria were used for males and females. Even in the presence of diabetes, cardiovascular risk factors were inadequately controlled in most patients. **Conclusion:** The concurrence of diabetes and other cardiovascular risk factors which constitute the metabolic syndrome is a common phenomenon in urban diabetic patients. It is possibly associated with hyperinsulinemia and gender.

[Key words] Diabetes mellitus; Cardiovascular diseases; Hyperinsulinism; Obesity; Hypertension; Sex

11. 瘦素受体基因变异与中国人肥胖的关系

瘦素受体基因变异与中国人肥胖的关系

［摘要］目的: 研究瘦素受体基因变异与中国人肥胖的关系。**方法**: 选择肥胖病人［体质量指数（BMI）≥30kg/m^2］和正常人（BMI<25kg/m^2）各50例, 抽提基因组DNA; 用PCR-SSCR技术筛查瘦素受体基因外显子1~7、12和18及内含子2的变异。**结果**: 在瘦素受体基因内含子2处发现有碱基改变（T→C）; 瘦素受体基因外显子18发现碱基改变（C→A）, 导致氨基酸由丙氨酸→天冬氨酸。**结论**: 瘦素受体基因内含子2发生碱基改变可能引起瘦素受体基因RNA剪切异常, 氨基酸改变可能影响受体的空间构象, 从而影响其功能。

［关键词］DNA突变分析; 瘦素受体基因; 肥胖; 中国人

Variation of the Human Leptin Receptor Gene In Obese Chinese Population

[Abstract] Objective: To investigate the relationship between the genetic variation of leptin receptor and obesity in Chinese population. **Methods:** Genomic DNA was extracted from 50 obese subjects [Body mass index (BMI) ≥30kg/m^2] and 50 normal individuals (BMI<25kg/m^2) by standard methods; primer pairs for PCR-SSCP specific to the genomic sequence of exon 1–7, 12, 18 and intron 2 were synthesized and PCR-SSCP was conducted to screen sequence variation. **Results:** Variations in intron 2 (T → C) and in exon 18 (C → A) were found and the latter caused an amino acid variation (Ala → Asp). **Conclusions:** The variation in intron 2 may result in abnormal splicing of leptin receptor gene RNA. The amino acid variation (A1a → Asp) in leptin receptor exon 18 may influence its conformation and function.

[Key words] DNA mutational analysis; Leptin receptor gene; Obesity; Chinese population

12. 一种新的流感快速诊断法

一种新的流感快速诊断法

目的：建立一种新的、简便、敏感、特异和重复性好的流感快速诊断法。**方法**：采集标本经成片 MDCK 细胞扩增，使细胞表面受体发生改变，借助植物素与细胞表面受体结合的严格特异性，通过不同光学显微镜来观察红细胞聚集现象，对测定标本做出判断。**结果**：新法与常规的 MDCK 细胞分离法符合率为 100%，一般 20h 内就可出结果；其敏感性比常规细胞分离法高 100~10 000 倍或以上；它既可用于临床上的流感快速诊断，又可用于流感监测；测定时最适红细胞浓度为 1‰，并测定结果不受人血型和豚鼠个体的影响。**结论**：新法简便、敏感、特异、重复性好，并具有多用途等优点。（出处:《中华实验和临床病毒学杂志》）

A Novel Test for Diagnosis of Influenza

Objective: To set up a novel,simple,sensitive,specific,repeatable and rapid assay for diagnosis of influenza. **Methods:** Monolayers of MDCK cells were inoculated with the specimens for amplifying viral, the feature of receptors on cell surface was changed by treatment of neuraminidases of influenza A and B viruses.Afterward, based on the lectin binds to receptors on cell surface with strict specificity, the phenomenon of red blood cell aggregation was observed under the conventional microscope. Finally, the tested result could be determined by the extent of red blood cell aggregation. **Results:** there was a complete (%) consistence rate (100%) for viral isolation between new and routine tests. In general, the result were detected with new assay within 20h. The sensitivity of new assay was over 100–10 000 times higher then than that of routine method. Meanwhile, the novel test could not only be used for rapid diagnosis in the clinic ,but also be used for influenza surveillance. The best concentration of red blood cells was 1‰ in the detection assay. The testing result was not effected by red blood cells taken from either different red blood cell type of human or different individual of guinea pigs. **Conclusions:** The novel method has several advantages: simple, high sensitivity and specificity, accurate and suitable for multiple purposes.

13. X 连锁性隐性非综合征型低频神经性听力减退的家系报道

X 连锁性隐性非综合征型低频神经性听力减退的家系报道

目的：探讨和分析低频神经性听力减退的遗传学因素。**方法：**从先证者出发，调查一个家系发病情况；应用 Cyrillic2.1 软件绘制系谱图；通过系谱图分析遗传学特征，通过临床检查分析疾病的表型特征。**结果：**调查现存家系成员 101 人，获得 43 人的临床听力学资料。43 人中有 6 人被诊断为低频神经性听力推荐，均为男性，年龄 10~36 岁；患者仅以听力减退为单一症状；临床表现特征为轻、中、重度及极重度听力损失，听性脑干反应均未引出，畸变产物耳声发射部分引出；患者发病年龄在 10~16 岁之间。**结论：**本研究发现了一个 5 代相传的遗传性聋大家系,遗传特征是以男性发病为主的 X 连锁隐性遗传。该家系的发现提示低频神经性听力减退可以是由遗传因素造成的。（出处:《中华耳鼻咽喉科杂志》）

A Report on a Large Family with X–linked Recessive Nonsyndromic Hereditary Low Frequency Neuropathic Hearing Impairment

Objective: To analyze the genetic causes of low frequency neuropathic hearing impairment. **Methods:** Using the network established by our institute, the proband of the low frequency neuropathic hearing loss pedigree was found. Then, investigation was carried out in the family from proband. Cyrillic 2.1software was set up to draw the pedigree and genetic characterization and phenotypes were analyzed in this family. **Results:** One–hundred and one alive family members were investigated and the clinic audiologic examination were performed in 43 of 101 individuals.Six of forty-three individuals appeared to be low frequency neuropathic hearing loss and all patients were ales without systemic disorders except hearing loss.The clinic phenotypes were mild, middle, severe and profound hearing loss with disappearing of the auditory brainstem response (ABR) and partial normal results of distortion product otacoustic emission (DPOAE) in the affected individuals.The onset of hearing loss was at 10–16 years old and the age of all patients was arranged from 18 to 26 years old. **Conclusion:** A large five generations family with hereditary low frequency neuropathic hearing impairment was found in our study. The genetic pattern in this family is male dominant x–linked recessive (XR) nonsyndromic hearing loss. Our findings suggest that some low frequency neuropathic disorders might be attributed to genetic factors.

14. 丁酸钠增强 U937 细胞凋亡敏感性的分子机制研究

丁酸钠增强 U937 细胞凋亡敏感性的分子机制研究

目的：探讨丁酸钠（NaBu）对细胞周期检测点效应及对 U937 细胞凋亡的敏感性。**方法**：以 U937-ASPI3K（ATM 阴性）、U937-pZeosv2（+）（野生型 ATM 基因）两种 U937 的变异细胞系作为细胞模型。用免疫沉淀及激酶活性测定 p38 MAPK、ERK1 的激酶活性。用免疫印迹分析 Bad 磷酸化灭活。**结果**：经 NaBu 预处理的 U937-pZeosv2（+）细胞经 ^{137}Cs 照射后，细胞凋亡敏感性呈 NaBu 剂量依赖性增强。这种增强效应可被 p38MAPK 阻滞剂 OLM 阻断，但不能被 p34cdc2 激酶的特异性抑制剂 ALP 及 CDK2 阻滞剂 CDK2-I 阻断。经 NaBu 预处理的 U937-ASPI3K 细胞经 ^{137}Cs 照射后，细胞凋亡敏感性进一步增强，这种增强效应可被 OLM 阻断。放射线可显著增强 p38 MAPK 激酶活性，抑制 ERK1 激酶活性；NaBu 预处理与放射线联用后，对 p38 MAPK 激酶活性的增强有极其显著的协同效应。放射线诱导 U937-ASPI3K 细胞 Bad 蛋白磷酸化灭活，在 NaBu 协同作用下，Bad 蛋白磷酸化灭活效应进一步增强。**结论**：NaBu 通过 p38 MAPK 激酶活性，增强细胞凋亡敏感性，该效应与 ATM 基因是否缺失无关，与 ATM 失活增强的细胞凋亡敏感性各为独立通路。（出处:《中华肿瘤杂志》）

Molecular Mechanism of Enhanced Apoptotic Response in U937 Cells Mediated by Sodium Butyrate

Objective: To study the effects of sodium butyrate (Nabu) on cell cycle checkpoint and the apoptosis sensitivity in U937 cells. **Methods:** Two mutant U937 cell lines, U937–ASPI3K (ATM negative) and U937–pZeosv2 (+)(ATM wild–type), were used as the cell model system.Immunoprecipitation and kinase assay were used to examine the p38 MAPK and ERKI kinase activities. Western blot was used to analyze the phosphorylation of Bad protein. **Results:** U937–pZeosv2(+) pretreated with Nabu exhibited enhanced apoptotic response in a Nabu dose dependent fashion upon ^{137}Cs irradiation, which could be abolished by olomoucine (OLM), a p38 MAPK specific inhibitor. On the other hand, Cyclin dependent kinase 2 (CDK2) specific inhibitor cdk2–I and p34cdc2/cyclinB inhibitor alsterpaullone(ALP) failed to block the effects of Nabu Similar results were also observed in U937–ASPI3K. The effect of irradiation on p38 MAPK and ERKI was strikingly potentiated by Nabu. Furthermore, inactivation of irradiated Bad protein via phosphorylation on serine 136 was also enhanced. **Conclusion:** Nabu is able to enhance the apoptotic response in U937 cells, which is mediated by p38 MAPK activation but not ATM status.

15. 乳腺叶状肿瘤的临床病理学研究

乳腺叶状肿瘤的临床病理学研究

　　目的：探讨乳腺叶状肿瘤的病理形态学特点、分类和诊断标准、与复发转移的关系及其临床意义。**方法：**采用回顾性分析的方法对 203 例有随访（6~372 个月）资料的叶状肿瘤作了详细形态学特征的分析和分类研究，统计学聚类判别分析。**结果：**良性 133 例（复发 28 例），交界性 42 例（复发 19 例，死亡 2 例），恶性 28 例（复发 18 例，死亡 15 例）。统计学分析结果显示，肿瘤生长方式、瘤细胞异型性、核分裂象计数和肿瘤性坏死所组成的变量子集分类错判率为零。以此 4 项为主，完善了病理组织学诊断标准。良性、交界性和恶性组间复发率、转移和死亡率差异均有显著性意义。肿瘤复发随术式的扩大而减少，2 次以上复发占 53.85%（35/65）。**结论**：此瘤可分为良性、低度恶性（交界性）及恶性三种类别。肿瘤生长方式、瘤细胞异型性、核分裂象和肿瘤性坏死是诊断此瘤并对其进行分级（分类）的重要依据。提示首次术式的选择的重要性，良性叶状肿瘤应选择肿物扩大切除术，对于复发的交界性和恶性肿瘤应作乳房切除术。（出处：《中华病理学杂志》）

Clinicopathological Study on Phyllodes Tumor of the Breast

Objective: To study the relationship between pathological features and classification criteria of the breast Phyllodes tumor. **Methods:** 203 cases of breast phyllodes tumor diagnosed it in 22 hospitals were analyzed and reappraised by a retrospective study. **Results:** 133 cases were benign, 42 cases were borderline and 28 were malignant. The follow-up (6 to 372 months) showed that 28/133 benign, 19/42 borderline and 18/28 malignant cases recurred, and 17 patients (2 borderline and 15 malignant) died. The statistic cluster analysis demonstrated that stromal cellar atypia, margin involvement, mitotic activity and tumor necrosis were retained in the variable group, and no error distinguish were showed. **Conclusions:** The breast phyllodes tumor can be classified as the following three types: benign, borderline and malignant. It is important to diagnose and classify the breast phyllodes tumor according to the involvement of tumor margin, stromal cellar atypia mitotic activity, stromal overgrowth and tumor necrosis. There are significant differences of 5 years survival rates recurrent rates and death rates between the benign, borderline and malignant breast phyllodes tumor. With wide excision the he recurrence of the tumor decreased suggesting that at broad excision is preferred for the benign tumor and mastectomy is indicated for recurred borderline and malignant tumors.

16. 牙槽骨垂直牵引成骨种植术的临床研究

牙槽骨垂直牵引成骨种植术的临床研究

　　目的：评价牙槽骨垂直牵引成骨技术在改善种植区域骨量中的可行性、临床效果及优缺点。**方法**：19 例因肿瘤切除术或外伤等原因造成重度牙槽突垂直向骨缺损（缺损均大于 10mm）患者接受了垂直骨牵引术，其中男性 15 例，女性 4 例，平均年龄 35 岁。常规行术前、术后及牵引前、后 X 线检查记录及取牵引器时直接测量牵引高度。安放牵引器 7d 后开始牵引，每日牵引 1mm 至设计高度。保留牵引器 2~3 个月，局麻下拆除牵引器，植入种植体。**结果**：19 例中 11 例已完成种植上部结构修复，已植入种植体尚未完成上部修复 6 例，共植入种植体 65 枚。19 例在牵引成骨后均形成理想新骨，平均新生骨的高度 13mm。牵引区意外骨折 2 例，牵引区感染 1 例，植入种植体后感染 1 例。**结论**：牙槽骨垂直牵引术是解决重度骨量不足的有效的替代方法。（出处：《中华口腔医学杂志》）

Clinical Study of Alveolar Vertical Distraction Osteogenesis for Implant

Objective: To evaluate the clinical result of alveolar vertical distraction osteogenesis for implant. **Methods:** 19 cases with severe vertical alveolar defects (more than 10 mm defect underwent vertical distraction procedure before implant placement. 15 cases were male and 4 cases were female. Preoperative, postoperative X-ray examination records and traction height is directly measured when the tractor is taken. After placing the retractor for 7d, it starts to pull, pulling 1mm. to the design height every day. Keep the retractor for 2–3 months, remove the retractor under local anesthesia, and implant placement. **Results:** 11 cases out of 19 had implant prosthesis. 6 cases had implant in the jaw but waiting for the prosthesis. Altogether 65 dental implants were placed, The study showed that new bone formed after distraction in all 19 cases. Average gained height of new bone was 13 mm. 2 cases did not receive further implant treatment because of cost problem. Complications: Unexpected mandible fracture in 2 cases, infection in 1 case. **Conclusions:** Alveolar vertical distraction is a good alterative for severe alveolar defects.

17. 结核分枝杆菌感染对人巨噬细胞离子通道及其调控元件转录表达的影响

结核分枝杆菌感染对人巨噬细胞离子通道及其调控元件转录表达的影响

为研究人巨噬细胞的离子通道及其调控元件是否参与了抗结核分枝杆菌感染免疫,利用表达谱芯片技术研究细菌感染后宿主巨噬细胞基因的表达情况。在全局表达谱分析的基础上,重点分析了离子通道及其调控元件的表达,并比较无毒株和临床分离有毒株在诱导离子通道及其调控元件表达方面的差异。结果表明,细菌感染影响离子通道及其调控元件基因的表达,涉及的离子通道包括钾通道、钠通道、氯通道、钙通道,差异表达的调控元件包括 G 蛋白、G 蛋白偶联受体、蛋白质激酶和磷酸化酶;临床株感染影响的离子通道及其调控元件较无毒株广泛和丰富。这些观察结果提示,离子通道及其调控元件参与了宿主细胞对感染细菌的免疫应答,有关离子通道及其调控元件在抗结核免疫中的作用有待进一步研究。芯片研究的结果为将来的研究提供了线索。(出处:《生理学报》)

Effects of Mycobacterium Tuberculosis Infection on the Transcriptional Expression of Human Macrophage Gene Encoding ion Channels and Related Regulatory Elements

Expression microarray was employed in this study to investigate whether the ion channels and their regulatory elements encoding genes participate in the immune response to Mycobacterium tuberculosis infection. The results of a virulent strain were compared with those of the clinically isolated strains, The data demonstrate that K^+, Na^+, Ca^{2+} and CI^- channels and their regulators, such as the G protein, receptor and second messenger, protein kinase and protein phosphatase were involved in the immune reaction, The clinical strain affected more types of ion channels and respective regulatory elements. The data provide clues for further scrutiny into the role of ion channels and related elements in the interaction between Mycobacterium tuberculosis and host macrophage.

18.　极端嗜盐硫解酶基因的克隆和氨基酸组成分析

极端嗜盐硫解酶基因的克隆和氨基酸组成分析

根据嗜盐菌（Halobacterium salinarum）NRC-34001 中硫解酶的基因序列信息，采用 PCR 技术从菌株 Halobacterium sp.ZP-6 中克隆了极端嗜盐硫解酶的基因并对此酶的氨基组成进行了分析。同非嗜盐硫解酶相比，极端嗜盐硫解酶不但含有较多的负电荷氨基酸，较少的正电荷氨基酸和强疏水氨基酸，而且同类氨基酸中的小氨基酸含量明显增高。这表明极端嗜盐硫解酶的嗜盐特性不单来自形成的分子静电屏蔽网和疏水作用的调节，且与分子表面张力减小密切相关。（出处：《微生物学报》）

Molecular cloning and amino acid composition analysis a halophilic thiolase gene

5' and 3' end sequence of acaBI gene as primers, the gene of halophilic thiolase from haloarchae, Halobacterium sp.ZP-6 was cloned and its amino acid composition was calculated. Compared with non-halophilic thiolase, the halophilic thiolase contains more negative charge amino acid less positive amino acid and less strong hydrophobic amino acid, and use preferably small side -chain amino acid. Those suggest that electrostatic screen, hydrophobic elect and surface tension all contribute to halophilic properties of thiolase.

19.　透明颤菌血红蛋白基因表达对金色链霉菌生长代谢的影响

透明颤菌血红蛋白基因表达对金色链霉菌生长代谢的影响

利用四环素抗性基因启动子在金色链霉菌中表达透明颤菌血红蛋白基因。在 $1m^3$ 发酵罐中研究了工程菌株的生长代谢特性。在溶解氧充足的条件下，透明颤菌血红蛋白表达，对金色链霉菌生长代谢未产生明显影响，工程菌株与参比菌株的生长代谢特性基本一致，工程菌株和参比菌株金霉素最终浓度分别为 22 905u/ml、22 896u/ml。在低溶解氧条件下，透明颤菌血红蛋白的表达，可促进金色链霉菌菌体生长、菌丝活力保持和金霉

素的合成：工程菌菌体浓度比参比菌株高 5%~10%，产物合成提高 11.4%。（出处：《微生物学报》）

Study on Effect of Vitreoscilla Hemoglobin Gene Expression on Growth and Metabolism of Streptomyces Aureofaciens

Vitreoscilla hemoglobin gene was expressed in S.aureofaciens through promoter of tetracycline resistance gene, Characteristics of S.aureofaciens growth and metabolism were studied in $1m^3$ fermenter. In high dissolved oxygen concentrations, expression of hemoglobin gene had little effect on growth and metabolism of S, aureofaciens and there were no obvious differences between engineering strain and control. The chlortetracycline of engineering Strain was 22 905 u/ml, and of control was 22 896 u/ml respectively. Under conditions of low dissolved oxygen, expression of hemoglobin enhanced growth, maintenance of energetic mycelium configuration and chlortetracycline yield of S.aureofaciens: the mycelium concentrations of engineering strain were more about 5%–10% and yield was more 11.4% than control.

20. 补阳还五汤抗缺氧再给氧乳鼠心肌细胞凋亡的实验研究

补阳还五汤抗缺氧再给氧乳鼠心肌细胞凋亡的实验研究

目的：观察含补阳还五汤的大鼠血清对缺氧 24h 再给氧 4h 后新生乳鼠心肌细胞凋亡的抑制作用及对一氧化氮（NO）含量的影响。**方法：**采用 Annexin V–PI 双标记方法（以流式细胞仪和 ELISA 法）检测细胞凋亡，以紫外分光光度法测定心肌细胞乳酸脱氢酶（LDH）释放水平,采用改良 Yu 方法测定 NO 浓度, 用 Ohkawa 法测定硫代巴比妥酸（TBARS）反应物质含量。**结果:** 补阳还五汤药物血清能显著抑制心肌细胞的凋亡及 LDH 释放,降低培养细胞上清液中 NO 和（TBARS）水平,其效应呈剂量依赖关系。**结论:** 补阳还五汤具有抗缺氧再给氧心肌细胞凋亡作用,其机制与清除氧自由基和 NO 特性有关。（出处:《中国中西医结合杂志》）

Study on Preventive effect of Buyang Huanwu Decoction on Cardiomyocyte Apoptosis Induced by Hypoxia Reoxygenation in Rats

Objective: To observe the preventive effect of rats' serum containing Buyang Huanwu Decoction (BYHWD) on cultured cardiomyocyte apoptosis of neonatal rat induced by means of 24 hrs hypoxia and 4 hrs reoxygenation, and to investigate its mechanism concerned with nitric oxide (NO). **Methods:** Myocyte apoptosis was detected by flow cytometry and ELISA with Annexin V–PI double labeled method. The lactate dehydrogenase (LDH) releasing level was measured with ultraviolet spectrophotometer. The NO concentration was determined by modified Yu method and the concentration of thiobarbituric acid response substance (TBARS) was tested by Ohkawa method. **Results:** BYHWD contained rats' serum could significantly prevent cardiomyocyte from apoptosis induced by hypoxia and reoxygenation. After hypoxia–reoxygenation, the NO, LDH and TBARS levels in the supernatant of cultured liquid treated with BYHWD were significantly lower than those in non–treated cultured liquid, the effect of BYHWD was dose dependent. **Conclusion:** BYHWD can prevent cardiomyocytes from apoptosis induced by hypoxia and reoxygenation, its mechanism might be related with oxygen free radical and NO scavenging produced during the hypoxia–reoxygenation process.

21. 恶性高血压与吸烟(资料性摘要)

恶性高血压与吸烟

将48例恶性高血压患者与92例非恶性高血压患者做了吸烟习惯的对比研究。初诊时已吸烟的恶性高血压患者有33例,非恶性患者34例,两者之间有显著差异。即使对男性患者进行比较,或将白人与黑人分别进行比较,这种差异也仍然显著。本研究表明:恶性高血压是一种与吸烟有关的疾病。

Malignant Hypertension and Cigarette Smoking

The smoking habit of 48 patients with malignant hypertension was compared with that of 92 consecutive patients with non–malignant hypertension. Thirty–three of the patients with malignant and 34 of the patients with non–malignant hypertension were smokers when first diagnosed. This difference was significant and remained so when only men or black and white patients were considered separately. Results suggest that malignant hypertension is yet another disease related to cigarette smoking.

22. 对一群体中饮食钾与血压关系的研究(资料性摘要)

对一群体中饮食钾与血压关系的研究

[摘要]对居住在加州南部一个以白人为主的社团中由685名20~79岁男女组成的群体进行的研究发现,根据24小时饮食史估算的饮食钾摄取量与调整了年龄因素的男女性

收缩压以及与调整了年龄因素的男性舒张压具有重要的负相关性。排除服用抗高血压药品物以及有明显高血压（血压>160/90mmHg）的人后，这些相关性依然存在；调整了其他各种饮食因素，包括酒精和钙的摄取后，这些相关性也还存在。在妇女中排除使用性激素者后，与血压的相关性提高了，说明激素状态可能是决定妇女血压的一个重要因素，而且可能会掩盖其他关系。这一发现支持了在各群体中饮食钾与血压有病因学关系。

[**关键词**]血压；饮食钾

Dietary Potassium and Blood Pressure in a Population

[**Abstract**] A population based study of 685 men and women aged 20 to 79 years old in a predominantly Caucasian community in Southern California found dietary potassium intake estimated from 24 hours recall dietary history to be significantly and negatively correlated with age-adjusted systolic pressure in both men and women and with age-adjusted diastolic blood pressure in men. These correlations remained after exclusion of persons taking antihypertension medication or those with categorical hypertension (blood pressure >160/95mmHg), and also persisted after adjusting for other dietary variables including alcohol and calcium intake. In women, correlations with blood pressure increased after excluding those taking sex hormones, suggesting that hormonal status may be an important determinant of blood pressure in women and may obscure other relationships. These findings support the etiological relationship of dietary potassium with blood pressure in populations.

[**Key Words**] Blood pressure; Dietary potassium

23. 恶性淋巴瘤伴有明显的嗜伊红细胞增多症（资料性摘要）

恶性淋巴瘤伴有明显的嗜伊红细胞增多症

一名60岁患低分化淋巴细胞型淋巴瘤的黑人，淋巴结呈全身性肿大，嗜伊红细胞明显增多。对嗜伊红细胞进行的大量研究发现，其形态与机能均属正常。患者经过可的松治疗后，肿大的淋巴结消失，周围血细胞计数恢复到正常范围。但仅维持了数月，原来的临床症状又复发。旋即开始全身性化疗。但疗效短暂。患者病情急转直下，最后死亡。本文综述了嗜伊红细胞增多症的发病机制和嗜伊红细胞功能研究的最新进展，并探讨了淋巴瘤与嗜伊红细胞增多症的关系。

Malignant Lymphoma Associated with Marked Eosinophilia

A 60-year-old black man with poorly differentiated lymphocytic lymphoma presented with generalized lymphadenopathy and marked eosinophilia. Extensive evaluation of the eosinophils revealed them to be normal morphologically and functionally. The patient responded to corticosteroid therapy with resolution of the lymphadenopathy and reversion of the peripheral blood counts to normal limits. Recurrence of the original clinical picture within months prompted institution of systemic chemotherapy. Response was transient, and the patient expired after an unremitting downhill course. Recent advances in our knowledge of mechanisms of eosinophilia and eosinophil function are reviewed. The relationship of lymphoma to eosinophilia is discussed.

第十一节　论文摘要的时态
（Tense of the abstract of dissertation）

　　写好医学论文英语摘要,时态的选用是一个关键问题。目前,国内出版的医学刊物的论文英文摘要大多数是依照其中文摘要逐字逐句翻译而成的,看似完整和清楚,但多数没有真正达意。尤其是在时态使用方面存在着严重的混乱现象。其实,在医学论文英语摘要写作中时态的使用是比较固定的。写作时应根据文章所要表达的内容,从时间的概念出发,考虑到不同时态所代表的不同意义,来正确地选用时态。本节选录了一些著名的刊物的英语摘要,并按时态类型进行了归纳说明。

1. 一般现在时

　　是撰写论文英语摘要中使用最广泛的时态,主要用于说明发表论文当时的情况,介绍本文的内容（包括本文的目的,这与表示研究目的不同）,表述作者的结论（因为科学的结论往往具有普遍真理的性质）等。

　　（1）介绍或陈述论文或实验背景

　　Four cases of plasma cell leukemia are reported that illustrate the variable immunotype of this disorder in contrast with the immunologic profile described for normal B-cell maturation and typical multiple myeloma (MM).

　　本文报告4例浆细胞白血病患者,并通过与所描述的正常细胞成熟的免疫分布和典型的多发性骨髓瘤进行对照来阐述这种疾病的不同免疫类型。

*　　　*　　　*

The present paper is designed to investigate the variation of pain threshold and electroacupuncture analgesia of rat, and to observe the immunohistochemical changes in spinal ganglion and dorsal horn of lumbar and sacral segment of spinal cord after extradural administration of capsaicin (100μg/rat).

对大鼠硬脊膜外注射 100μg 辣椒素后，观察其痛阈，电针镇痛效应以及腰骶段脊髓后角和脊神经节的免疫组织化学变化。

（2）简单通报研究内容

A male with thyroxine-binding globulin (TBG) excess and an autonomously functioning thyroid adenoma is presented. The problem of diagnosing hyperthyroidism in the presence of TBG is discussed. The utility of the thyrotropin-releasing hormone test (TRH) is emphasized.

本文报道 1 例甲状腺素结合球蛋白过多症的男性患者合并有自主功能甲状腺瘤，讨论了 TBG 过多时甲状腺功能亢进的诊断问题，本文还着重介绍了甲状腺素释放激素试验的使用价值。

*　　　*　　　*

We describe two patients who developed pleural fibrosis after treatment with practolol.

我们报道 2 例患者应用普拉洛尔继发胸膜纤维化。

（3）表述作者结论

These changes suggest that, in the absence of luminal acid, small organic acids, such as aspirin and acetic acid, may have complex effects on the ironic conductance of surface cell membranes without altering intracellular pH.

这些变化表明，在缺乏巴比妥酸的情况下，小分子有机酸，如乙酰水杨酸和醋酸对表面细胞膜的铁电导可能具有复杂的作用,但不会改变细胞内的 pH 值。

*　　　*　　　*

It is proposed that nonspecific ulcers of the colon should be managed conservatively.

我们建议,非特异性结肠溃疡应保守治疗。

（4）一般现在时还常用在定语从句中作客观规律、真理等内容的补充说明。

These metallic changes were explained by the reduction of redox state which accompanies ethanol oxidation.

随乙醇氧化而发生的氧化还原状态的减少解释了这种代谢变化。

*　　　*　　　*

We investigated the regulation of GAP43 gene expression in PC12 cells, which are believed to resemble precursor cells of the adrenomedullary lineage.

我们调查了 PC12 细胞中 GAP43 基因表达的调控,据认为它与肾上腺髓质系的前体细胞相类似。

2. 一般过去时

用以介绍实验的材料和方法,叙述研究过程,陈述实验结果。随着医学科学技术的发展,以及它与人类的健康息息相关,现在的医学论文更偏重于客观地报道实验的材料和方法,研究过程以及实验结果,又因为这些科研或实验全部都是在过去进行的,因此,一般过去时也是撰写论文英语摘要中使用较广泛的时态之一。

（1）陈述研究目的:陈述研究目的过去一向被认为是应该

用一般现在时来表述，但现在人们大多用一般过去时来表述。

The purpose of this study was to consider the time interval for periodic mammographic screening for breast cancer.

本研究旨在探讨定期乳腺 X 线摄影检查乳腺癌的间隔时间。

*   *   *

The purpose of this study was to determine whether enterocyte transplantation could be used to correct a specific genetic metabolic defect.

本研究旨在确定肠细胞移植是否可用来矫正特异性遗传代谢缺损。

（2）介绍实验材料和方法

Total hepatic protein synthesis was measured in vivo with a flooding dose technique, and the production of total secreted proteins, albumin, complement component C3, and serum−mucoid fraction was measured in perfused livers of septic rats that received one of three different solutions infused intravenously…

肝蛋白合成的总量是用溢量（flooding-dose）法在体内测定的，总分泌蛋白、白蛋白、补体 C3，以及血清黏蛋白成分的产生是在经静脉注射了 3 种不同溶液中的 1 种的脓毒症大鼠肝脏中测定的……

*   *   *

Patients were randomized into groups of 25 patients each: a control group and a heparin group. Changes in the venous blood flow were monitored using Doppler ultrasonic flowmeter.

将病人随机分成 2 组（对照组和肝素组），每组 25 人。用多普勒超声流量计监测静脉血流变化。

（3）叙述研究过程

The smoking habits of 48 patients with malignant hypertension were compared with those of 92 patients with non-malignant hypertension.

作者将48例恶性高血压患者与92例非恶性高血压患者作了吸烟习惯的对比研究。

（4）陈述实验结果

This protocol resulted in a considerable reduction in toxicity, as compared with that described in previous studies, without compromising the efficiency.

本次记录的结果是,与前几次研究所描述的结果相比,毒性明显减小且不危及效能。

*　　　*　　　*

End-diastolic and mean PCP were significantly higher over the left than right ventricle at high [(20.3 ± 1.0)mmHg] and middle levels [(13.7 ± 0.9)mmHg] of left atrial pressure.

左动脉压在高电位[(20.3±1.0)mmHg]和中电位[(13.7±0.9)mmHg]处,左心室的末端舒张压和平均PCP明显高于右心室。

3. 将来时

表示以后要做的工作或预期的结果。

（1）表示以后要做的工作

As greater clinical correlation is obtained, the usefulness of thyroglobulin determination will increase.

随着甲状腺球蛋白测定与临床的相互关系日益密切,其诊断价值也将提高。

（2）表示预期的结果

In both cases bacteria were grown from the bile and it is to be hoped that bile culture will be recorded more commonly in future in cases of this interesting condition.

这2例胆汁中均培养出细菌。可以预料，今后在遇到这一引人注意的疾患时，胆汁培养会更加普遍。

4. 现在完成时

说明论题的发展背景，指出该项研究尚存在着空白的领域，或强调该研究项目已经完成。

The toxic effects of acute or chronic use of alcohol on cerebral and hepatic function have long been recognized, but it has been thought that the heart was not similarly affected.

暴饮或长期饮酒对脑及肝脏的毒性作用久已为人们所知，但人们一直认为对心脏并无类似影响。

5. 过去完成时

通常被用来补充说明实验或研究之前的一些必须交代的情况。多用于定语从句中。

Serological effectiveness was outstanding: all of those who had been seronegative became seropositive following either two intradermal or subcutaneous infections given one month apart.

血清学效果显著：血清反应阴性的人皮内或皮下每月一次，注射2次后都变成阳性的了。

医疗机构名称用语

X-线申请单	application for X-ray examination
X-线技师	X-ray technician
X-线室	X-ray room
X-线科医师	roentgenologist
儿科	department of pediatrics
儿童医院	children's hospital
入院处	admission office
卫生员	health worker
卫生医师	hygienist
门诊部	out-patient department (O.P.D.)
门诊病人	outpatient
口腔科	department of stomatology
少生优生	fewer and healthier births
内分泌科	department of endocrinology
引产	induced/artificial abortion
中心检验室	central laboratory
中医科	department of traditional Chinese medicine
化验员	laboratory technician
手术室	operating room, operating theatre
手术台	operation table
计划生育	family planning information consultation
咨询服务	consulting services

内科　　　　　　　　　　department of internal medicine

内科医师　　　　　　　　physician

水疗科　　　　　　　　　hydrotherapy room

中国心理卫生协会心　　　Board of Psychological Assesment, China
　理评估专业委员会　　　　　Mental Health Association

化验申请单　　　　　　　Application for laboratory examination

处方　　　　　　　　　　prescription

电疗科　　　　　　　　　electrotherapy room

皮肤科　　　　　　　　　department of dermatology

皮肤科医师　　　　　　　dermatologist

平均住院日数　　　　　　average of hospital staying days

中国心理卫生协会中　　　Board of Chinese Child Mental Health,
　国儿童心理卫生专　　　　　Chinese Mental Association
　业委员会

出诊　　　　　　　　　　to visit a patient at home, to pay a home
　　　　　　　　　　　　　　visit, to make a house call

出生证　　　　　　　　　birth certificate

出院处　　　　　　　　　discharge office

主管医生　　　　　　　　physician in charge, doctor in charge of
　　　　　　　　　　　　　　case

主治医生　　　　　　　　attending physician, visiting physician

世界卫生组织心理社　　　WHO Collaborating Research Centre for
　会因素成瘾行为与　　　　　Psychosocial Factors, Drug Abuse
　健康合作中心　　　　　　　and Health

主任医生　　　　　　　　chief physician

外科　　　　　　　　　　department of surgery

外科医生　　　　　　　　surgeon

牙科医生　　　　　　　　dentist

生化检验室　　　　　　　biochemical laboratory

优生优育　　　　　　　　bear ard rear better children

产科医师	obstetrician
产科医院	maternity hospital, lying–in hospital
男护士	nurse, attendant, male attendant
死亡证	death certificate
血库	blood bank
血清检验室	serological laboratory
传染病科	department of infectious disease
传染病院	infectious disease hospital
传染科医师	doctor for infectious disease
光疗科	phototherapy room
节育	contraception, birth control
耳鼻喉科	E.N.T. /otorhinolaryngological department
耳鼻喉科医师	E.N.T. specialist, otorhinolaryngologist
创伤外科	department of traumatology
护士	nurse
护士办公室	nurse's office
护士长	head nurse, the sister
护理部主任	matron, senior nursing officer
护理部	nursing department
住院医师	resident
住院总医师	chief resident
住院部	in–patient department
住院病人	in–patient
住院治疗	hospitalization
戒毒康复病室	Detoxification and Rehabilitation Treatment Centre
会计	accountant
会诊	consultation of doctors
诊断书	medical certificate
助产士	midwife

初诊	first visit
妇科医师	gynecologist
妇产科	department of obstetrics and gynecology
泌尿科	department of urology
泌尿外科医师	urological surgeon
肿瘤医院	tumour hospital
附属医院	affiliated hospital, hospital attached to a medical college/university
实习生	intern
实习护士	student nurse
供应室	supply room
医生办公室	doctor's office
医嘱	doctor's advice
夜班	on night duty
转院	transfer to … hospital
转院证	certificate of transference
胸科医院	chest hospital
胸外科	department of chest surgery
××科主任	… head/director of the department of
总务科	general affairs section
挂号员	registrar
挂号处	registration office
治疗室	therapeutic department
育龄夫妇	married couples of childbearing age
神经外科	department of neurosurgery
神经外科医师	neurosurgeon
神经科	department of neurology
骨科	department of orthopedics
骨科医师	orthopedist
临床检验室	clinical laboratory

复诊	further consultation, subsequent visit
查房	go the rounds, make one's rounds, do one's rounds
院长	superintendent of the hospital, director of the hospital
独生子女	only child
消毒室	disinfection room
候诊室	waiting room
配膳室	diet preparation department
细菌学检验室	bacteriological laboratory
值班	on duty
病历	case history
病历室	record room
病床	hospital bed
病床周转率	turnover rate of hospital beds
病室服务员	ward servant
病室女服务员	ward maid
病房	ward
病假证明	certificate for sick leave
麻风病院	leprosy hospital
麻醉师	anesthetist, anesthetist
麻醉学家	anesthesiologist
清洁员	cleaner
流行病科	department of epidemiology
流行病医生	epidemiologist
教学医院	teaching hospital
矫形外科	department of orthopedic surgery
矫形外科医师	orthopedic surgeon, orthopedist
结核病院	tuberculosis hospital
结核病医师	doctor for tuberculosis

理疗科	department of physiotherapy
理疗科医师	physiotherapist, physiatrist
停尸室	mortuary
领药单	a requisition for drugs
晚婚晚育	late marriage and late child bearing
药房	pharmacy, dispensary
药房主任	head of the pharmacy
药剂士	assistant pharmacist
药剂师	pharmacist
换药室	dressing room
眼科	department of ophthalmology
眼科医师	ophthalmologist
营养部	nutrition department
综合医院	general hospital
精神病院	psychiatric hospital, mental home, mental hospital, mental institution, mental health clinic
精神病医生	psychiatrist
精神病人	mental patient, lunatic
精神病学	psychiatry
整形外科	department of plastic surgery
整形外科医师	plastic surgeon
避孕措施	contraceptive measures
避孕套	sheath
避孕器,避孕剂	contraceptive